Who Moved My Magnet?

PETER GIBSON

For Patti & Skip
Stay well !
[signature]

AMT PRODUXIONS LLC

WHO MOVED MY MAGNET?
How you are moved like a magnet through the medical maze
And the amazing history behind the construction of that maze

Published by AMT ProduXions LLC
12460 Crabapple Road, Suite 202 #377
Alpharetta, GA 30004
1 888 WOMBAT1

Manufactured in the United States of America

Library of Congress Control Number: 2005910074

Who Moved My Magnet?
Gibson, Peter
ISBN 0-9719991-9-8
ISBN 978-0-9719991-9-8

1. Health   2. Children's Books   3. Self Help
How you are moved like a magnet through the medical maze.
And the amazing history behind the construction of that maze

Edited by: Claudia McCormick
' Illustrated by: John Foster
Book design: Jill Dible

To the lifesaving work of traditional medicine.

And to the life-preserving work of alternative medicine.

ACKNOWLEDGEMENTS

Isabelle, my dear wife, thank you for the incredible support you have given me to write this book. Alexander, my special son, I know you will be happy to see other kids, and their parents, enjoy the WELLNESS WOMBATS™ as much as you have.

The St. Louis team: Cathy McCredie, Joe Sartori and John Foster. How can I ever thank you for the four years of encouragement and support? Cathy lit the way Joe helped edit the way and John patiently sketched ways to visualize it so that readers of all ages would have fun with the ideas that the WELLNESS WOMBATS™ *Who Moved My Magnet?* spawned.

"First a good book," my editor said. Well, Claudia McCormick of BookWriters, your name is on this one. Thank you for not letting me put out anything less than a good book.

Creating text for the WELLNESS WOMBATS™ to burrow around in has been fun. I want to recognize the people who supported what I was creating: Helen Dumba, Diana and Steve Long, Robin Rider and Anja Stas-Rider, Bruce and Sharon Moon, Robyn Stalson, John Knight, Betty and Jim Starnes, Dr. Bob Burdette, Joyce Rennolds, Jack and Sheri Clarke, Danny and Amy Barcelona, Werner and Elaine Beiersdoerfer, Bart and Brigitte Vantieghem, Peter Janssens, Carine Bourgeois at The Roswell Tea House, Frank and Gabriella Wagman, Teresa Weems, Bobbie Christmas, Paul Qualey, Maureen May, Ruth Kent, Kalpana Murthy and Crystal Frantz. I appreciate every nurse, medical, and wellness practitioner who freely gave me insights about their profession to incorporate into this book as well. And finally, I thank every parent, and child, who inspired me to support their commitment to their family's health by writing this book. I hope *Who Moved My Magnet?* helps others see how becoming WELLNESS WOMBATS™ makes staying out of the medical maze fun.

FOREWORD

In a wonderful, creative and entertaining way Peter Gibson has enlightened children, teenagers and adults to the importance of taking personal responsibility for good health and becoming a Wellness Wombat, someone who inspires others by word of mouth testimonies to take care of their health. He carries us through the history of medicine and explains so well how over time it has pulled us in many different directions. He explains how we have been manipulated and mislead into thinking that if we don't do what mainstream medicine says then we don't have a chance of survival from many diseases. For years people have been scared to death by a doctor's diagnosis and prescription for toxic, poisonous drugs in the name of "healing".

The "health care" system as we know it today is really the "sickness care" system. We spend more money than any nation on earth for health care and yet the American people are some of the sickest on the planet. We rate low in the statistics of good health in comparison to many much poorer countries. We spend more and more in the name of good health but continue to get sicker. What's wrong with this picture?

Insurance companies continue to approve multi millions of drugs and surgeries for clients but won't pay for educational classes to teach people how to personally take better care of their health so they won't need drugs, surgery and other expensive traditional treatments. It is sad that illness has become a multi-billion dollar "business" and that so many people are getting rich off others being sick, but this is the world that we currently live in. I believe that we can transform this negative energy into positive when we decide, one person at the time, to take total responsibility for our health and to do whatever it takes to become as healthy as possible.

It isn't easy to go against what the doctor says because so many people believe that it's the doctor's way or no way. In 1999 when I was told by my doctor that if I did not do surgery and chemotherapy that I would die in six months to a year I did a controversial thing by going against my doctor's recommendations and looking for a more natural way of helping my body heal itself. Some of my friends and family couldn't understand why I wouldn't do exactly what my doctor said and they tried to influence me to change my mind. It didn't work because I had personally seen relatives and friends diagnosed with similar diseases try conventional medicine only to have their diseases and tumors return to the same or another part of the body. Then they would get cut on again, have another body part or tumor removed, be bombarded with more toxic poisonous drugs and still they would not heal. This conventional method is all about treating the symptoms, but not much at all about true healing of the body. This is not the way to good health.

Even with my doctors, friends and family members in disagreement, I made my own decision to change my thinking patterns, get on a healthy nutritional program, detoxify my body, learn to deal better with stress, exercise more, heal the old emotional stuff and miraculously my body did what it was intended to do all along, it healed itself. Within 6 months of my changing my lifestyle, my tumors were gone; I was 70 pounds lighter, with no more arthritis, low energy, depression, allergies, or severe headaches. Without even realizing it, that's when I became a Wellness Wombat. I decided to open The Living Foods Institute in Atlanta, Georgia so I could spread the word and teach as many other people as possible that they too could take back their power and their health in a natural way. Without knowing it, I was a living breathing Wellness Wombat! My first book, The Living Foods Lifestyle, tells the story of how I went from a victim, much like Rick in this story, to a hero like Warren and Wanda. By healing my own health challenges I was able to teach and inspire others to do the same. I'm not the only one who has done this. There are many Wellness Wombats out there with inspirational testimonies sharing incredible stories and positive results. This is good, but we need more. You can never have too many Wellness Wombats!

Until I read Peter's book I didn't know what to call myself, a teacher, a minister, a healer or a helper. Until now I have just been a woman with a mission to tell others what worked for me and have encouraged people to try it for themselves to see if it will work for them. Now I discover through "Who Moved My Magnet" that I am a Wellness Wombat! When we follow the basic laws of nature and truly honor ourselves by taking good care of our bodies, we will be rewarded with good health.

There are two systems of health care available in America: traditional western medicine and alternative medicine. The first is the world of the American Medical Association; medical doctors who practice by the book, and who inadvertently align themselves with the multibillion dollar pharmaceutical industry. Traditional medicine is superb when it comes to surgery, emergency, and trauma, but there's no question that alternative medicine works better for most everything else.

Diseases like cancer, heart disease, rheumatoid arthritis, asthma, headaches, allergies, sinusitis, gastrointestinal problems, fibromyalgia, lupus, MS, Parkinson's, depression, obesity, drug and alcohol addictions are better helped with alternative therapies. I find it interesting to hear the term "alternative therapy" applied when talking about natural ways of healing as if these were a secondary way of helping the body and one that should only be tried if all else fails. Most alternative therapies including herbs, essential oils, colon cleansing and detoxification with natural foods have been around long before traditional medicine as Peter describes in his book. It isn't the new alternative, it is the real deal, something that has been with us a long time, we just forgot about it as the medical maze pulled us into its game! It is the way that I believe the body was intended to be supported for good health, with everything coming from natural resources and good old Mother Nature.

Alternative medicine has a lot to offer you, but our government is ignoring this and funds are not being sufficiently allocated to study alternative ways. We should all be asking, "Why?" I believe that most of us will come up with the same answer, MONEY. Sickness is a big business. We do not have to fall victim to this. We can think for ourselves. We can gather information and get the education about how to properly take care of ourselves. We can gather all this information and that will be wonderful, but none of this will help us until we actually put the principles to practice for ourselves. It's not just in the learning what to do, it's the doing it!

Some think of advances in medicine like lasers or a new drug or surgical procedure as the latest, greatest way to health. We have a hard time believing that the simple choices we make each day like what we eat, how we think, if we smoke, or drink too much, if we do or don't exercise, meditate or relax are the real key to our success in manifesting health or our failure by manifesting disease. Good lifestyle choices can make a powerful difference in our health and well being, even in our quality of life and longevity.

Peter has created a story that is easy to read and understand. The Wellness Wombats are sure to become the next action figures for good health! Wanda, Warren and Doc are the heroes of today. They are the ones not afraid to speak out to educate others like Rick in this book, and the millions of other Ricks out there that are drawn into the maze of traditional medicine like a magnet. It is so easy to get swept into that maze. Peter has cleverly taken us on a journey through history to see how this has happened, where it has gotten us, and now what we can do about it.

This is a book that I believe will help everyone who is ready to become empowered to think for themselves, to ask questions, to investigate and find out how to become responsible for their own health rather than looking to someone else to fix it for them. It's a story that will appeal to all ages and make the journey to good health fun!

Whether or not you agree with everything in this book is not as important as drawing your own conclusions based on the data and evidence that Peter has presented. It is powerful information intended to get us thinking for ourselves.

I applaud the time, commitment and dedication that Peter has given this project so "Who Moved My Magnet" could come to fruition. I am happy to know that I am a Wellness Wombat and that there are many others like Peter and possibly you too who are a Wellness Wombat now or wanting to become one.

Don't wait another day to get on the band wagon for good health. Reap the rewards and then tell everyone. Read this clever book, and then share it with others. You too can be a Wellness Wombat. We need millions of them. It all starts with one person and that person is you. Don't try to fix the rest of the planet until you do something about yourself first. This book is a great place to start!

Rev. Dr. Brenda Cobb
Founder and President of Living Foods Institute
Author of *The Living Foods Lifestyle,*
Colon Cleansing For Optimum Health,
Get Started Now Towards Better Health,
101 Raw and Living Foods Recipes,
The Living Foods Lifestyle Training Manual.
www.livingfoodsinstitute.com
800-844-9876
Atlanta, Georgia, November 21, 2005

CONTENTS

Who Moved My Magnet?
is part of the WELLNESS WOMBATS™ Series

Diagnosis:

The Tale Behind This Tale

WHY DOES MEDICINE HAVE SO MUCH INFLUENCE ON HOW you manage your health?

How did it come to be so big and acquire so much pull and power over you?

What is it that draws you to the emergency room, or to the doctor, and makes you think about medicine first whenever you feel sick? It can't be the drab buildings, the long waits, the short answers the doctor gives you, the side effects of the drugs he prescribes, or the insurance and billing paperwork. It can't be the way you are dehumanized by revealing hospital gowns, busy all-knowing doctors, and technology you don't understand. It can't be the intimidating maze of corridors that all lead to rooms where you, as a patient, will be expected to bare yourself and the personal details of your medical history.

Oh, yes, medicine wants to know all about your medical history. But, did you ever wonder about its history?

Who Moved My Magnet? reveals it. It walks you, the health-conscious consumer, through medicine's unhealthy history and uncovers a record of events that just may make you sick.

Warren and Wanda, two wellness advocates along with Ed, a medical doctor fed up with the ways of the medical maze, meet their sick friend Rick in Quackers Juice Bar. To help Rick see how he fell into the medical trap and how he was conditioned to believe that medicine was the healthiest course for him, Warren dissects its history. To represent those people who took a stand against how that structure was built and fought for the right to manage their own health and not have it managed for them, Warren invents the Wellness Wombats.

A Wellness Wombat is in the word of mouth business all the time (hence the acronym WOMBAT), and willingly shares the benefits of wellness over sickness and self-care over managed care to anyone who asks. He practices positive health habits and learns how to move his own magnet so that he can avoid being moved like one into the medical maze. He doesn't want to be caught in the flux, or the repetitive cycle of unhealthy patterns he thinks medicine practices.

Medicine, or the maze in which it operates, is important; hospitals are full of brilliant, talented people who save lives. If you need a broken bone fixed, or heart surgery, go to the hospital. But, if you are like most people today, you are nervous about how traditional medicine profits from the influence it has over you and your day-to-day health concerns and, even more important, what its motivations are. You consider holistic medicine instead; whether it's massage, homeopathy, Tai Chi, yoga, meditation, chiropractic, or even organic food, you seek alternatives. You are not sure when you will find the time or make the changes to practice them, but you want them.

Who Moved my Magnet? gives you the incentive to change. It caringly delivers the message that you must pull away from the influence that the medical maze holds over you and experience, first-hand and for yourself, how much fun taking responsibility for your health and moving your own magnet can be. It's a message I constructed after spending over twenty years taking care of my own health and ten years consulting with others about better ways to manage theirs.

I wrote *Who Moved My Magnet?* to help you see what I saw when I began to question how medicine got to be the force it is today, and why it so easily leads and bleeds the Ricks of the world. To help you see how influenced by and reliant upon medicine you may have become. To prompt you to think about how much responsibility you may have given up for your health. To make you ask: "Who is moving my magnet? Who is really in charge of my health?"

I created the Wellness Wombats so that kids, and their parents, would see that being well is far more fun than being sick. If our children are not healthy, how can we expect society to be? The Wellness Wombats can make practicing a healthy lifestyle fun, so that it is something everyone will want to do and not be ashamed to do.

Taking care of your health and convincing your children to take care of their health shouldn't be an inconvenience; it should be an enjoyable part of your everyday life that ultimately leads to a more fulfilling and longer life. You can't afford to be sick, and it's swell being well. The Wellness Wombats not only help you pull away from the ways of the maze and practice healthier ways; they make that journey fun.

Prologue:

The Quacks Charter
Twenty years ago

"THERE YOU ARE, WARREN," DOC SAID, LOOKING UP FROM his table by the window of The Cordial Café. "Have a seat, my friend."

Warren Burrows grabbed the wooden chair across from Doc and sat down. "Good to see you again. Say, I've been thinking about your idea and I like it. It's way ahead of its time."

Doc's large hands cradled his mug of ginger tea. "It's just what Atlanta's Little Five Points community needs: a bigger juice bar and health food store. I've got my eye on that old tavern next to Witch Hazel's Magic Shop. It's been vacant for a while now. I need your help with the name, though." Doc pointed at the open book he was trying to keep balanced between his knee and the table. "I read something in here that I think I can use. It's a name that sums up how willing we health-nuts and granola-munching tree huggers are to mock ourselves."

"Unlike medicine, you mean, that is not?" Warren replied, sipping on his green tea.

Doc chuckled. "You're the history buff; you know alternative medicine has always been discredited by traditional medicine, so it hasn't taken itself as seriously about the power it holds to help heal others. You and I both know that there are as many quacks over there;" Doc gestured toward Hickory Medical Clinic, visible through The Cordial Café's window, "in that part of town, as there are over here in this part of town, to keep that debate going for a while."

"Quack is such an interesting word, isn't it?" Warren said with an authoritative tone. "It comes from the Dutch word quacksalver for someone who sold questionable remedies. Most people have conflicting opinions about what it means. Medical doctors see alternative practitioners as quacks and alternative practitioners see medical doctors as quacks."

"So, let the people decide who the quack is," Doc responded. "Anyway, here's what I found in this book." Doc began to read. "In 1542, King Henry VIII passed what came to be known by skeptical and jealous doctors as the 'Quacks Charter.' It allowed herbalists and people who were not licensed or certified as doctors to treat illnesses on the surface of the body with plasters, poultices, and ointments. In England many alterative therapists still practice under this charter today."

Warren lowered his voice to make his point. "They still call them quacks in the States. Besides, Henry VIII was a keen amateur herbalist, so it's no wonder he did what he could to protect other herbalists from the greedy doctors of the day who viewed anything they didn't approve of as witchcraft or snake oil. So, how does this tie in with a name for your health food store? Are you going to call it 'Quacks'?"

Doc laughed. "No, I'm going to call it 'The Quackery'. And I'm going to call the juice bar next door, 'Quackers'. What do you think?"

"I think it's great. You've got enough supporters of holistic medicine who choose self-care over managed care in this neighborhood to fill the place. And in about twenty years, when the rest of Atlanta comes around to organics and all the stuff we've been doing to stay healthy, you might attract that crowd too."

Doc raised his mug of tea. "Then here's a toast," he said, "to our health, the health of our community and the health of this great city."

Warren tapped his teacup against Doc's favorite mug and looked around the Café. "To the quacks in here and the quacks over there," he said, glancing through the window toward Hickory Clinic. "I hope they all shop at The Quackery and eat at Quackers Juice Bar one day."

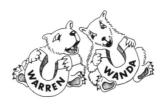

A Walk in the Park

"SUMMER IS OVER," WARREN SAID, AS HE TOSSED A FEW LEAVES in the air. "And the year two thousand five will be gone before we know it." He turned his boyish-looking face toward his wife. "I don't feel like I've aged a bit."

Wanda brushed the falling leaves out of her hair. "I don't either," she replied. "Isn't it great? We're both approaching fifty and still have the energy of most thirty-year-olds." Her slender but strong arm held the iron gate at the park entrance open to let an elderly couple through. "So, tell me about your wombats."

"Wellness Wombats," Warren stressed, his athletic frame following Wanda's wiry one through the gate, "they are going to make taking care of your health a lot more fun."

Wanda looked over her shoulder. "A healthy lifestyle is something more people realize that they have to take responsibility for practicing on their own these days; they can't afford to be sick."

"People can't afford to eat the junk food Main Street menus offer either, or consume the medications the medical maze has conditioned them to take," Warren replied. "They have to change their ways and seek out alternatives. They know medicine performs miracles; they know that if they treat their body well it will perform miracles too. But most people just don't see taking responsibility for their health as a walk in the park."

"Well, medicine doesn't encourage them to repel unhealthy habits and attract healthy ones, now does it? Wanda asked walking briskly beside Warren now. "Medicine has built a healthcare model based on sickness, not on wellness."

"A model I think the Wellness Wombats can help people avoid being drawn into."

"And how will Wellness Wombats do that?" Wanda asked.

"You're the marketing expert. You told me the first thing they taught you in marketing class was the power of word of mouth, right?"

Wanda gave him a questioning look. "Yes?"

"And that everyone's in the word of mouth business."

"Everyone is," Wanda confirmed, "even if all they do is recommend a good movie or share the name of a restaurant."

"So when people share the benefits of good health, they become Wellness Wombats," Warren replied enthusiastically. "We're Wellness Wombats because we manage our own health. We don't depend on medicine to manage it for us. We avoid negative health habits and practice positive ones. We respect and listen to our bodies, strive to avoid stress, live a healthy, balanced, life, and share the benefits of that lifestyle with others."

Wanda stopped walking. "Okay," she said, "go ahead: explain."

Warren picked up a stick and scratched six crooked letters in the gravel on the path. "WOMBAT is an acronym," he said. "Look." He pointed the stick at each letter and slowly spelled it out. "WOMBAT: word of mouth business all the time. We're all in it."

"Clever! So, if I pass on the benefits of my experience pursuing positive health habits, or the stories you always share about the unhealthy history behind the construction of the medical maze, I become a Wellness Wombat?"

Warren grinned. "And if you dig health enough, wombats dig burrows, you know, you'll share the benefits of that lifestyle with others."

Wanda took her husband's hand and they started walking again. "Charming," she said. "Just like you. People are going to love this especially at Charter Spa and Wellness Center which, thankfully, I can take a day off from managing today. It's a fun way to get your message across. I can see you creating little toy Wellness Wombats one day to help guide people out of the medical maze."

"Good idea. Plush little toys to lead kids away from Main Street's fast food chains and the drugstores that lead them there." Warren's hearty laugh filled the crisp fall air.

"So, when did you come up with this?" Wanda asked.

"Last week. I was telling our son bedtime stories."

"You two and your stories; I know about the project on Australia Joey brought home from school last month and about the wombat tales you've been spinning him at night. He told me his friends teased him about his last name being Burrows, too, when they discovered that wombats burrow to create the maze of tunnels they live in. So, the stories you told him gave you the idea for the Wellness Wombats?"

Warren's laugh simmered down to a chuckle. "That and the fact that our friend Rick called last week, desperate to meet for lunch today, so he could talk about his experience in the hospital. I was looking for a fun way to help him as well. To get him to listen for a change, to what we we've been trying to tell him about his unhealthy ways."

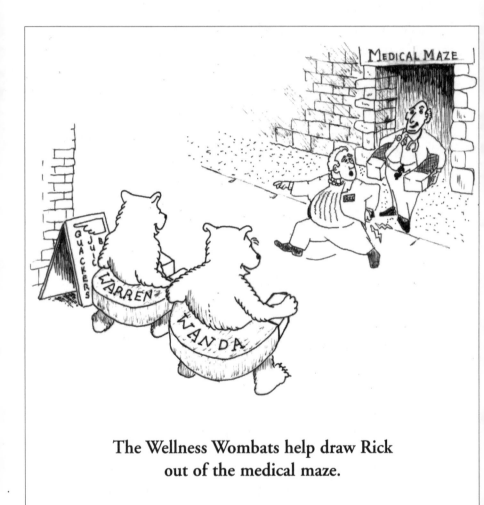

**The Wellness Wombats help draw Rick
out of the medical maze.**

"How they lead him into the medical maze, you mean?"

Warren threw the stick away. "Doctors ask their patients about their medical histories. I wonder if it occurred to Rick to ask his doctors about theirs; about medicine's history, I mean. Before he signed consent for surgery forms and put his health in medicine's hands."

The September breeze gently blew Wanda's black hair across her face and she brushed it aside. "We warned him. We tried to wake him up to how unhealthy his habits were. He looked pretty sick the last time he came in to Quackers."

"I can't believe it's been twenty years since I sat down at The Cordial Café with Doc to help him pick that name," Warren said, leading his wife past the duck pond. "All this talk about repelling negative habits and attracting positive ones reminds me of how much we tease Rick about being moved like a magnet through the medical maze."

"I'm always teasing Joey about that," Wanda replied, "whenever I need to remind him why we eat healthy foods every day. I know he gets it because he came home from school one day telling me how our body is like a magnet, and how all matter generates electromagnetic energy. It's what keeps our body running."

"The same energy that the Chinese refer to as chi," Warren said above the sound of the blowing leaves, "energy that circulates just as the field of a magnet does; energy that needs to be fueled and fed properly." He smiled. "Joey knows he has to eat well because, like a magnet, he attracts and puts out energy, and the energy he puts out is only as good as the energy he takes in to fuel his body."

"I know, junk in junk out. It's no wonder so many kids today are tired and overweight. They keep fueling their bodies with the wrong stuff. If Rick had listened to us and eaten at Quackers

Juice Bar more and on Main Street less, he wouldn't have been moved like a magnet into the medical maze as fast as he was."

"Rick ended up in that maze," Warren said, "because traditional medicine's magnet, or influence, is stronger than alternative medicine's magnet. Medicine has deliberately conditioned, moved, and manipulated the Ricks of the world to rely upon it and to not look for alternatives. But that's changing, because people want to know more about alternative care, not medical care, today. People are looking at our field of medicine again, and are willing to be drawn into it because they don't trust the way medicine operates. That's where the Wellness Wombats come in. They will help draw people like Rick away from the maze and toward healthier ways and will weaken the influence medicine has by making the mention of prevention and its practice fun."

Warren looked in the direction of Hickory Clinic visible across the park. "Well, Rick is overweight, overwhelmed, and was over there. Ed, our rebel doctor friend that works at Hickory Clinic, told me Rick was under a lot of stress. He worked six-day weeks managing his crews installing fiber-optic cable. He had no time for himself or his family."

"His back gave out, right?"

"That's what finally put him into the hospital, but his lifestyle and diet provoked it; breakfasts at the gas station, drive-thru lunches, and snacks all day."

"So, tell me the story," Wanda said tossing her hair back from the blowing wind. "How did you come up with the Wellness Wombats?"

Warren's warm storyteller voice kicked in. "Okay, here's the story: A busload of tourists, on their way to Sydney, stopped on the side of the road to eat. Warren wombat and Wanda wombat, which usually sleep most of the day so they can graze at night, were basking in the sun at the edge of their warrens and could see the bus."

Wanda giggled. "Now that's cute. You named them after us. I bet Joey was thrilled."

"He was, about the names, the moral of my story, and that wombats with their short tails, short legs, and cuddly appearance are as cute as koalas. Anyway, the tourists, unlike the wombats who eat grass, shrubs, herbs, and other natural foods, stuffed their faces with the fast food they had picked up earlier: unnatural food, at least in the eyes of the wombats."

Wanda glanced at her husband. "Let me guess; they left a bunch of trash behind."

"Correct," Warren replied. "Styrofoam containers, dirty napkins, plastic cups, paper bags, snack bar wrappers, soda straws. You name it. And leftover fries, burgers, and cookies. You might say the unhealthy side effects of their unnatural diet."

"So, what did the wombats do?" Wanda asked. "I mean, what did Warren and Wanda do?"

"Wombats scrounge for food, just like any other animal, so they waddled over to it and began to eat from the trash the tourists left. The food was convenient, so they ate it, but they paid for it later. Remember, I'm making this story up for Joey. Wombats are herbivores, they eat grass and chew on tree roots, and they are not supposed to eat fast food leftovers. Anyway, the result of this irresponsible act was that they got sick and suffered for a few days. But, they also woke up to how unhealthy it was to eat those foods and get off their natural diet."

"Just what we've been telling our friend Rick Weaver."

"I know," Warren said. "Anyway, Warren and Wanda wombat began to tell others about their unhealthy experience, to help them learn from what they had done. They begged other wombats to avoid the temptation of discarded fast food, or leftovers from campers or hikers. And told them that they would live longer if they had the discipline to go look for grass, bark, shrubs, and herbs, which is their natural diet, and not get hooked on the manufactured taste, or convenience, of unhealthy and unnatural foods."

"That's the moral of the story, then? To take responsibility for what you eat, for how you live?"

"Yes, but, more importantly, to pass that message on to others. To become a Wellness Wombat and use word of mouth to pass on the benefits of your health habits. Without preaching and acting like you have the only alternative," Warren stressed. "You see a Wellness Wombat is not a zealous evangelist but, if asked, will share the benefits of wellness. He doesn't have to become an advocate like us. We actively promote the benefits of a preventative holistic lifestyle."

"That's my husband: my charismatic, storytelling husband. I love your idea and I love your wit." She gave him a quick kiss on his cheek. "And I love that you're fit instead of flabby. So, what happened next? How did our wombats become Wellness Wombats?"

"To prevent their kids, or their joeys as young wombats and kangaroos are called in Australia, from inheriting the unhealthy habits the tourists had displayed, Warren and Wanda wombat gathered other wombats from around the burrow. They shared the lesson they had learned: that it was better to eat whole, natural foods and be healthy than be enticed by food manufactured by humans and be sick."

"So, by sharing the benefits of what they had learned, they became Wellness Wombats?"

"That's right," Warren said enthusiastically, "and their community, their warren, benefited too. By reminding their fellow wombats to dig their health by taking responsibility for it, and by word of mouth to share the benefits, Warren and Wanda wombat helped keep other wombats responsible too. They weaved wellness through their warren, stopped poor health habits from spreading, and prevented other junk-food toting tourists from infecting yet another community. They taught their fellow wombats to respect nature's ways and question modern ways."

"To avoid the medical maze. I love it," Wanda, said. "It has potential."

Warren bowed to his wife, grinned mischievously and said, "Thank you," and resumed walking again. "I think Wellness Wombats can answer the question parents have about how to make eating food that's good for you fun. They're going to make my favorite topic, medicine's unhealthy history that I share with people every chance I get, more fun, too. Telling Joey his bed-time story prompted me to turn medical history into a series of ten short stories with my Wellness Wombats woven in. Now even Joey can understand why he needs to seek alternatives to the medical maze. I spent the last two weeks trying my stories out on him. He loves them. I think he's excited about being a Wellness Wombat and helping his friends at school to eat healthily, too."

"Oh gosh," Wanda exclaimed, "you've already got our eight-year-old telling his friends he's a Wellness Wombat?"

"You'll find out when you pick him up from school. Right now I want to try my stories out on Rick. He loves to hear me talk about the mess medicine is in. He's stuck in his ways and won't listen to the benefits of ours, but he might listen now. To the Wellness Wombat version of medicine's history, I mean."

Wanda hesitated. "You've missed his company, haven't you?"

"I've missed our verbal sparring."

"If Rick's overweight office manager Di Beatties hadn't dragged him in to Quackers, he'd never have bothered with us," Wanda said.

"And we never would have become friends."

"Debating buddies, you mean. He's the perfect foil for you, and you know it. You're friends with Rick Weaver because he got your attention when he called you a quack the first time he came into the Juice Bar. You've been trying to show him how consumed he is by the unhealthy habits we avoid ever since."

Warren kicked up some gravel. "I want to help him even more now after those unhealthy habits put him in the hospital. I like Rick. Not just because he challenges our lifestyle and mocks the way we manage our health, but because he's curious about how we do it.

As for the quack label, medicine stuck that one on us years ago so it wouldn't stick on them. They knew what they were doing. I don't think Rick, as sick as he looked when Di Beatties brought him in, knew why he was calling us quacks, or what that quackery might save him from one day."

"From a medical model that's not working," Wanda said, "one that fewer people can afford to put their trust in these days."

Warren smiled in agreement. "I know, but our gripe with medicine isn't with what *they* do. Doctors perform miracles every day. It's how they strive to suppress what *we* and our wellness practitioner friends do. Besides, it's what we do and how big that doing is becoming that traditional medicine fears today."

"And what is it exactly that we do?"

"We're Wellness Wombats, remember? We help people like Rick avoid the medical trap and alert them to the ways of the maze."

"In the hope they'll get on a healthier path, an alternative one?"

"Well, Wanda, as we both know, there are quacks in both fields of medicine. That's why we encourage people to walk the middle path of self-care and self-responsibility, a path that let's them choose traditional or alternative medicine without being misled by either. Sadly," Warren sighed, "medicine would rather people didn't have that choice."

"I'll bet Rick wished he'd chosen an alternative path right now and listened to us, instead of criticizing us every time we got together."

"It was fun debating our differences," Warren replied, "but I think our little taunt: Take Better Care; Avoid Medicare, may have more meaning to him now."

"We'll find that out when we see him at Quackers. I'm just glad he's out of the hospital." Wanda brushed a pine needle off Warren's shoulder. "Speaking of debating differences, how did it go at The State Capitol this morning? And tell me about your meeting at Hickory Clinic, too."

Warren slipped into his storytelling voice again. "Mr. Warren Burrows, business owner and distributor of software for computerized storage of medical records to hospitals, has been invited back to Hickory Clinic for a second meeting, and a chance to sell his system."

"That's great!"

"Thanks. Being a medical history buff paid off. The hospital administrators were impressed with the perspective I have of their industry; my presentation made the other sales presentations seem stale."

Warren took his wife's hand and squeezed it gently. "As far as my work at The State Capitol, I love the debates but it's a slog fighting for the rights of consumers who would rather pass kidney stones than digest the stuff in the bills that legislators are passing. Bills that restrict people's rights to choose alternative healthcare over traditional care."

"One day," Wanda said hopefully, "people will catch on to how their rights to manage their own health have been eroded by the bills you're fighting against being passed. People are losing the right to manage their own health, and they're too busy to see it."

"No, they allow their rights to be taken away. The comforts the medical maze offers them became more attractive than the disciplines that staying out of the maze demand. Anyway, Senators like Perry Stalsis and Ian Sincere don't help," Warren complained. "Every time a House Bill designed to protect health rights, not take them away, makes it to committee, Perry Stalsis blocks it. He doesn't even get off his favorite stool at The Capitol Tea Room to do it. He uses the phone."

"When did our governing bodies inoculate the public with the mantra: you don't have to be responsible for your health?"

"Oh, about 1885, actually, when Otto von Bismarck of Germany began the socialist experiment with medicine. In 1933, Roosevelt's New Deal set Americans up to expect the government to be the great provider and, in 1965, Lyndon Johnson sealed the deal. He gave us Medicare so that people wouldn't have to care, for their health that is!

"Tell it like it is why don't you?"

Warren opened the gate at the end of the park for Wanda and stepped aside. "You know I always do. Let's go. Rick will be at Quackers soon. I'm eager to hear what happened to him at Hickory Clinic."

Wanda pressed her agile form against Warren's muscular frame. "Eager to invite him to be a Wellness Wombat, you mean," she said as they crossed Clifton Road's tree-lined, pedestrian-friendly street and headed toward Quackers Juice Bar.

"Eager to see how far he got moved through the medical maze, actually," Warren admitted. "We told him he'd get moved like a magnet through the medical maze if he didn't stop scoffing at our ways while mindlessly pursuing his own. Well, he got moved all right. Let's go see how far!"

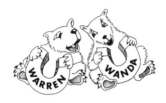

Quackers Juice Bar:
Atlanta

"AAH, QUACKERS. I LOVE THIS PLACE," WANDA SIGHED, AS SHE admired the patched brick interior and original stone fireplace visible from the entrance.

Warren had read the sign on the door a hundred times, but he read it out loud again as he held the heavy oak door it was posted on open for his wife. "Welcome to the health maven's haven, the gathering point for the health conscious community and its practitioners; where freedom of choice is the only alternative."

Wanda stood aside to let some customers leave. "Go on," she said patiently.

"I love this thing," Warren said as he kept reading. "In 1542 quack doctors from prestigious universities in London demanded that King Henry VIII protect the city they were practicing medicine in from uneducated pagan healers - other quacks. Instead, he scolded his doctors for being so greedy and passed The Quacks Charter, making it legal for herbalists to heal people, too." Warren spoke louder when he got to the inscription at the bottom of the sign. "The doctors didn't realize that King Henry was a keen amateur herbalist."

"You're not going to read the rest?" Wanda asked, starting through the door.

"Quackers Juice Bar welcomes quacks from traditional and alternative medicine. If you choose the healthy path, then walk this way. Make us your alternative choice," Warren finished as he followed Wanda through the door and over to the crowded bar.

"Hello there! How are my quack friends doing, today?" Doc said, greeting his two most popular customers from behind the horseshoe-shaped bar.

"Good to see you, Doc," Wanda called cheerfully, watching her footing as she made her way across the uneven wood floor.

Doc's six-foot frame and large hands dwarfed the juice blenders he was tending. "So, how goes the war against quackery? And what's the latest at The Capitol? Is the Medical Board going to pass that House Bill restricting how alternative therapists can treat their clients? Is the Food and Drug Administration going to shut me down for selling quack remedies and force me to take vitamins off my shelves?"

"Same old stuff, my friend," Warren said loud enough to be heard above the noise of the blenders, the bar crowd, and the chatter drifting through the entrance to The Quackery Health Food Store next-door. "People who don't protect their rights to manage their health allow others to take those rights away."

Doc picked up his tray full of red beet-based juice filled glasses. "Be right back, guys."

Wanda and Warren took a seat at their favorite end of the bar. "Hey Cal," Warren said, "good to see you."

Cal Ceum looked up from the Naturopath News he was reading. "Warren and Wanda Burrows. Good to see you," he said calmly. "I heard your verbal sparring buddy Rick Weaver is sick, the one with the back problem."

"Yeah, we spoke on the phone last week and arranged to meet here for lunch today," Warren replied.

Calvin chuckled. "I hear he just got out of hospital. Maybe he's ready for alternative care now."

"Judging by the size of the medical mob from Hickory Clinic in here today, he's not the only one," Wanda observed.

Calvin sipped his green barley juice. "Oh, those nurses and doctors, you mean? Heck, they're as fed up with medicine as anyone. Being in here is the healthiest alternative they've got."

"So, how's the nutrition business treating you, Cal?" Wanda asked.

Calvin put his journal down. "I'm swallowed up with orders, but that may not last if new directives on vitamins and dietary supplements are made law by this new bill, and doctors get to prescribe what people can swallow and I don't."

"You're right to be concerned," Warren agreed. "A similar law has already passed in Europe under the guise of protecting public health; medicine may pass it here too, without informing the public whose health they are supposed to be protecting."

"They're protecting the medical business," Wanda said. "The medical maze, I mean. Making sure it stays healthy instead of us."

"If it becomes law, it will paralyze my business, and Doc's Health Food store next door," Calvin said. "Medicine will dictate at what potency a vitamin or supplement should be prescribed or sold in stores and people who now buy higher milligram vitamins from me will be forced to go to a traditional doctor to get them."

"These are the kinds of bills I fight at The State Capitol all the time," Warren said angrily, "bills that restrict consumers from freely choosing how they manage their own health."

"Calvin sighed. "Medicine is doing what it's always done, protecting its own turf; just as Wanda said."

"But the drug industry is only seventy-five years old, Cal; natural cures have been around for centuries," Warren insisted. "They are not just protecting their turf; they are disputing the fact that they need nature for their turf to grow."

"I know," Cal sighed. "So, what have you been up to? You look tired."

"Oh, I spent another morning at The State Capitol fighting bills pending legislation that take away the health rights of citizens too busy to even care about their health, that's all."

"And what about you Wanda, you look ten years younger than you are as always. How are things at The Charter Spa and Wellness Center?"

"Where we're voting for your constitution?" Wanda said, anticipating Calvin's next remark. "Buying that place was the smartest move I've made, Cal, thanks."

Warren turned back toward the bar. "Hey, Doc, is the magnetizer on?"

"I'll check," Doc leaned under the bar and flipped a switch. "It is now."

"Tell me what that thing does again," Calvin asked.

Doc lined up three empty juice glasses for his next order. He turned the blender off. "It energizes you, Cal. The electromagnetic fields it generates affect nerve cells, muscle cells, and soft tissue." Doc poured juice into the glasses, picked them up and left.

Warren explained. "The magnetizer restores our connection with the magnetic energy that our bodies need, Cal.

Concrete and steel encased buildings block natural magnetic fields from reaching us. Every office should have one; people would experience a lot less in the way of stress if they did."

"Ah, yes. I read somewhere that all mammals have magnetic crystallite in their heads," Calvin responded. "It works as a guidance system when they're migrating or something like that."

"Haven't horse trainers been using pulsating electromagnetic products on their animals' injuries for years?" Wanda asked.

"That's right. Our all-knowing government approved of them as bone growth stimulators to treat slow healing fractures," Warren commented before turning his head and boyish face back to look at Calvin. "Hospitals are attracted to magnets too; they use magnetic pulses on patients who are suffering from depression. Transcranial magnetic stimulation, they call it."

"Hospitals? Did I hear someone say hospitals?"

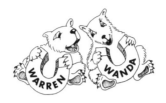

The Doctor is in

WANDA TURNED AROUND AND SHIELDED HER EYES FROM THE spike of sunlight beaming through the tall antique window frames. "Ed," she said, looking up at a tall slim man wearing designer glasses and sporting a well-trimmed beard. "Good to see you again."

Doctor M. "Ed" Esin greeted Warren and Wanda with his 'I'm your doctor and you're in good hands' smile. He sat down on the bar stool next to Warren. "Good to be in here for lunch again, instead of at Hickory Clinic where healthy food isn't even on the menu. So, where's Rick?"

Warren moved some cheese around on the plate of bar snacks in front of him. "He's running late," he said popping a piece of goat's cheese into his mouth.

Ed's smile waned briefly. "If Hickory Clinic gave him the jolt I think they did, then I'm not surprised he's late."

"Warren's going to shake him up some more," Wanda announced, "with his ten-stage take on how the medical maze Rick got caught in was built."

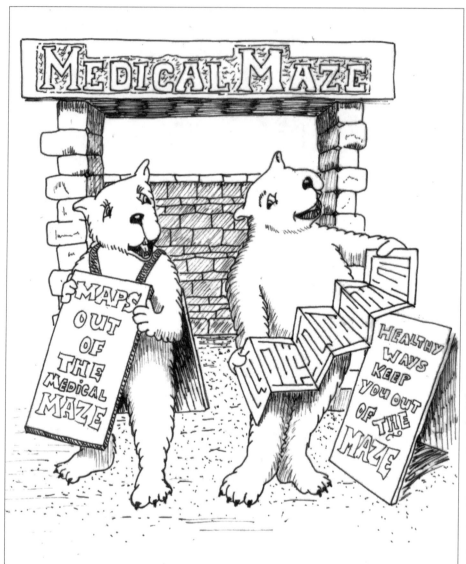

Healthy ways keep you out of the maze.

"That'll wake him up faster than the sound of a metal bedpan hitting the floor. Be careful, though," Ed warned. "I like your revealing ten stages about medicine's unhealthy and manipulative history, but not everyone is ready for them."

"Which is why I've created the Wellness Wombats," Warren exclaimed.

Ed peered over his glasses. "Wellness Wombats. What will you think up next?"

"I told Joey a bedtime story recently about a busload of tourists on their way to Sydney. They stopped on the side of the road to eat. Warren and Wanda wombat were sunbathing beside their warrens; they watched the tourists eat junk food and leave trash behind. The wombats ate from it, got sick, and learned a huge lesson about how healthy their habits were, and how unhealthy modern man's were."

"So, we want to use the Wellness Wombats as a fun way to get the word out about wellness now, and to share the benefits of a healthy lifestyle," Wanda said. "Joey's been doing a project on Australian animals at school. The wombat is one of his favorites."

"The word WOMBAT is an acronym for word of mouth business all the time," Warren explained.

"Word of mouth works. It's how I've built my reputation." Ed sipped on the Barely Barley Juice that Doc had placed in front of him. "I like your Wellness Wombat idea. It makes being healthy sound like fun. Get the parents or the kids behind it, to talk about how tired they are of the sickness model and how badly they want a wellness model, and the trust they've lost in traditional medicine may get transferred to alternative medicine again."

Wanda was excited. "I think this will help people see that changing their health habits can be fun. I'm going to share the Wellness Wombat idea with family members at my Spa. A lot of moms are looking for ways to get their kids interested in health."

"Rick Weaver is interested in his health," Warren responded, "but, like most people he has no real incentive to change his ways and stay out of the medical maze. I think I created the Wellness Wombats because I got tired of repeating my 'healthy ways keep you out of the medical maze' message to Rick and others I meet like him. Rick finished up in the medical maze anyway. Maybe the Wellness Wombats will get his attention and help guide him out of the maze to healthier ways."

"They'll deliver your message, but in a more appealing way," Ed suggested.

"Hey, Ed, don't you think Warren would make a cute wombat?" Wanda teased.

"I know this sounds hokey, and it's probably why my friends call me Educated Ed, but I read something about the Hebrew name for the wombat meaning, 'pocket teddy bear.'" Ed's smile broadened. "So, Wanda, what makes you think Warren would make such a great wombat?"

"Wombats have large brains, so they are smarter than they look. And, like Warren, they are physically strong and mentally determined. They are also full of energy and love to play. Warren would make a great Wellness Wombat!"

"A little large for a pocket teddy bear, but it certainly has a great ring to it," Ed said stroking his beard. "You know, traditional and alternative medicine could use your Wellness Wombats to make healthcare more fun. They might keep more parents and children out of the medical maze. Wombats could help them decide which type of care to pursue if and when they needed to as well; traditional medicine, struggling to gain the public's trust by medicating it; or alternative medicine, striving to earn public trust by educating it. Besides, I'd bet that you'll find more people willing to listen to a Wellness Wombat promoting a movement than a zealous health nut provoking a revolution."

Warren grinned. "I'm glad you like it, Ed. There'll be resistance, though. Medicine will want to combat the wombat. And repel it from the walls of the medical maze."

"Naturally," Ed replied, helping himself to the goat cheese. "Doctors have been trained to defend the ideas they've inherited, and to not be open to new ones. But don't worry; more doctors are questioning medicine's ideas and its quackery these days."

"My question right now is," Wanda said, reaching for her share of the cheese, "what does a Wellness Wombat stand for? We must define that before the people who want to embrace the idea to become one, do."

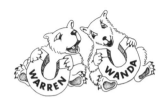

Warren's Wombats

"TIMELY QUESTION," WARREN REPLIED, EAGER TO SHARE HIS idea. "A Wellness Wombat takes responsibility for his own health. His incentive is to stay out of the medical maze and not depend on medicine to manage it for him. A Wellness Wombat moves his own magnet."

"And shares with others the benefits of his lifestyle, right?" Wanda said.

"Right, but I don't expect all those who become Wellness Wombats to promote its benefits the way we do but, if asked, they should by word of mouth share their stories," Warren stressed. "People become a true Wellness Wombat when they pass wellness on to their community.

I don't expect Rick to become an advocate like we both are. We want to break the patterns of medicine's unhealthy history that suppress people's freedom to choose alternatives. We want a more integrated medical model. If we can inspire Rick to become a Wellness Wombat, then he might embrace some of the same alternative practices that keep us out of the medical maze. He might respect and listen to his body more, avoid stress, and live a more balanced life."

"Then I'm with you Warren," Ed proclaimed. "I'd love to see Rick Weaver, if he'd get here that is, become a Wellness Wombat."

Wanda chuckled. "I'd love to see other people like Rick become Wellness Wombats. Like the people we see at the park stuffing down a fast food burger and drinking soda from their water bottles. They run to keep fit but skip right past the how to be healthy part."

Ed laughed. "Ha! That sounds like medicine's dilemma. In its quest to be fiscally fit, it's skipping right past the healthy part, too."

"It's not just the medical model that has us in a dilemma, Ed," Warren responded. "Corporate financial scandals, church leader scandals, school violence scandals, medical blunder scandals, and now drug scandals are in the news. HMOs and State social programs are going bankrupt, health-care costs are skyrocketing, employee benefits are dwindling, and public trust is fading. Everything needs a makeover."

Ed agreed. "Medicine certainly does. I'm tired of the power its corporate bean counters wield, of its arrogant and compla-cent hospital culture, and the medical messiahs it nurtures. A lot of my colleagues are, too. We aren't supposed to even suggest alternative therapy. We have to promote the medical way because of pressure from the drug companies that support us. But we're sharing the benefits alternative medicine provides more and more because we no longer trust in the ways of maze."

"Then your colleagues are Wellness Wombats too!" Warren claimed.

Ed cradled his juice glass in his hands. "Yes, and medicine is worried. Instead of integrating complementary medicine, it's watching its profits get chiseled away by alternative medicine. Because it's shackled by its own history, it is in no hurry to mimic that which it opposes most. It's burdened with the job it has inherited which is to suppress anyone from practicing anything that can't be defined as medicine."

"Did you say practice?" Warren queried. "Eighty percent of medicine is guesswork."

"I know," Ed said, "but give medicine some credit. It may be trying to resuscitate its old male-dominated ways by defending the crumbling walls of its maze, but it's coming around. Medical schools teach more about nutrition now. Medicine has revived the bedside skill of patient observation, or bedside manner, that William Osler was famous for around the turn of the twentieth century. It encourages massage and energy work; and 'quack' practices like blood sucking leeches to remove toxins are coming back. I won't even talk about the incredible opportunities mapping the human genome holds. Medicine is finally waking up."

Wanda was getting restless. "Consumers are waking up too, Ed, and they are all potential Wellness Wombats. More people are eating organics, buying whole foods, and cooking at home. People have to wake up if they want to free themselves from their reliance on medicine's proud science and its demanding allegiance to outdated incantations like, 'see your doctor', or, 'take your medication.' People need to learn how to take responsibility for their health, how to move their own magnets."

Wanda leaned forward suddenly and put both hands on the bar. Her energy was evident. "Wait. That's it! We've talked to Rick before about being moved like a magnet through the maze called healthcare, haven't we?"

"Yes, many times," Warren shot back. "How positive health habits can keep him out of it and negative habits pull him into it."

"So, why don't we have our Wellness Wombats hold magnets? The magnets will signify that they have taken responsibility for their health, by practicing positive habits, and can't be influenced by the power medicine holds over them anymore. They can't be moved, like a magnet is moved, through the medical maze. By carrying a magnet they provoke the question: Who's moving yours?"

Warren was enthusiastic. "I like where you're going, or given the current state of medicine should I say flowing?" he joked, "but it only works as a metaphor since opposite poles of magnets attract. If we perceive medicine as a negative place to be, or the negative pole of a magnet, our positive habits, or the positive pole of the magnet, would draw us into the ways of the medical maze."

Wanda was standing up beside her barstool now. "That's fine; I'm only using the magnet as a metaphor, as a symbol of how people are influenced and moved like one."

"I'm with you," Ed said. "Go on."

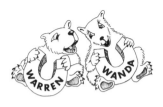

Wanda's Current Cure

WANDA'S WORDS TUMBLED OUT LIKE PILLS SPILLING OUT from a knocked over prescription bottle. "Advocates of positive health habits, like us, are strong enough to resist being drawn into the healthcare maze. We refuse to be influenced by the food, drug, or medical industries. We seek alternatives to their all consuming ways."

"Hmm," Ed mumbled, as he took his glasses off and cleaned them with his smiley faced tie, "but the Ricks of this world are another matter. They are easily influenced, easily led."

"Easily misled, you mean," Warren said quickly. "They consume what is marketed to them. They are so easily moved that medicine moves them like magnets into their maze: a maze people who don't take care of their health gladly enter because they see it as their only choice when they are sick."

Ed put his glasses back on and adjusted his tie. "Once they are inside the maze, they are intimidated by the knowledge and technology that medicine wields; they submit, in a haze, to the glaze of their ways. They unwittingly surrender their independence and their dignity right along with it."

"But Wellness Wombats can stay out of the medical trap," Wanda declared, "and keep others out of it too, by practicing and encouraging others to practice positive health habits so they won't get caught in the current of medicine's care."

"And moved like a magnet into the medical maze." Warren reached for his juice. "I love it. It flows, like the field of a magnet flows."

"Wanda's cure is very current," Ed teased. "But if we want medicine's influence to draw fewer people into its maze, then more education is needed. People can become better if they are better educated first. They have to be willing to change their ways if they want to stay out of the maze. And if they hear Warren's version of the history of medicine they'll want to change how much they depend on it for their health pretty quickly. The draw, if you'll pardon the pun, which your Wellness Wombats have, is their ability to make learning more about healthy ways a fun way to stay out of the medical maze."

"You're right, Ed. A lot of people who want to manage their own health and not have it managed for them are already applying positive health habits. They've bothered to learn how important those basic habits are, and tried to make sure they and their kids eat and live well. But the Wellness Wombats are still important because they can help everyone, at whatever level, become better educated about their health and inspire them to manage their own healthcare by seeking alternative care. They can help the Ricks of this world and their kids see that learning how to manage their health is fun."

Warren put his hand on Wanda's arm. "The magnets you want our Wellness Wombats to hold, are they horseshoe-shaped magnets? The same shape as Doc's bar?"

Wanda took a piece of pineapple from the snack tray. "Yes."

"Good, then your idea flows," Warren said firmly. "We take the two Wellness Wombats, Wanda and Warren wombat from the story I told Joey, and have each one clutch a horseshoe-shaped magnet. The magnet will symbolize the decision they have made to take responsibility for their health, to move their own magnets." Warren paused for a second. "Even better, the two wombats can hold their magnets together to form the letter 'W', for Wellness."

"And use the 'W' as the first letter for both wellness and wombats. Perfect!" Wanda cried. "That's the logo, then. That's our marketing tool."

"Great idea," Ed agreed.

"I can't wait to share this with Rick," Wanda said.

"You won't have to," Ed said. "He just walked in."

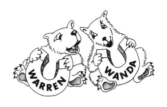

Rick Is Back

WARREN MET RICK'S OUTSTRETCHED HAND WITH BOTH OF his and smiled. "Rick, my friend, we're so happy to see that you are finally out of that hospital. How do you feel?"

Rick's belt had retreated under his belly; he tried to pull it back up. "Good to see you all," he said quietly, panting slightly as he joined his friends at the bar. "Thanks for coming. I never thought I'd be this glad to see you all again."

"Do you want to sit down?" Warren asked.

Rick's smile was more of a grimace as he gripped the back of his bar stool. "No, thanks, I'd rather stand. It's my back you know. The doctor told me not to sit for too long."

"We missed you Rick," Wanda said. "You've been in the hospital. What happened?"

"Yeah," Rick said. "Hickory Clinic: back surgery. It wasn't pretty, but it got me thinking. Your comments about my lifestyle have been on my mind more than I care to admit."

"It took back surgery to get your attention?" Warren asked. "A few more weeks of ribbing from us could have done that."

"And saved you from medicine's clutches," Dr. Ed added.

Rick held up both hands as if he were stopping traffic. "I know, I know. You warned me every time I came in here. My overfed, undernourished, stress-filled lifestyle was making me sick. I gave too much time to my cable company job and not enough to myself and my family. You were right. I should have listened. My bad habits put me in the hospital."

"It's tough being at the mercy of medicine's marvels, isn't it?" Ed said dryly.

"Yes, Ed, pretty humbling," Rick replied. "One day I was free to live my life the way I chose; the next I was wondering if I'd live."

"Because you chose managed care instead of taking care," Wanda declared. "You put your health in someone else's hands."

"I almost died in there," Rick said in a hush. "When you get that close to losing your life you suddenly appreciate it more. Now I know how valuable my health is and how badly I want to stick around to see the grandkids one day."

"Tell us what happened," Wanda whispered.

"That's why I wanted to meet with you all, to tell you what happened, and figure out why it happened to me."

"It was your back, right?" Ed said.

"Yeah," Rick sighed. "My beautiful but hyperactive wife, Rita Linn, asked me to move some furniture. Bless her, but she should have known better than to ask someone with a history of back problems, especially someone who never exercised. That's why I loved my job. I didn't lay cable; I managed the crews who did. My back would never have let me lay cable. Anyway, I bent over and twisted my back and it gave out on me. Later my right leg hurt, too. I didn't pay much attention to it at first, until I couldn't sleep, sit, or bend that is."

"Sounds painful," Wanda said, frowning as if she were experiencing the pain herself.

"It was," Rick said, grabbing a piece of rice cheese from the snack tray and putting it on a napkin. "I lay in bed for days and cried day and night. Rita Linn was concerned, of course, and told me to go to the hospital. I put it off. She insisted, and called our doctor and told him the pain pills weren't cutting it. He immediately told her I needed surgery. We had insurance, but when I heard the word surgery I got scared."

"And now you're scarred," Warren said.

"I hope it wasn't unnecessary. Back surgery is one of the most unnecessary procedures in medicine."

"Oh, thanks for telling me, Ed. My doctor didn't mention it, nor did the doctor on staff at Hickory Clinic. He put me through an MRI and found a ruptured disc pinching a nerve, so he confirmed the diagnosis and recommended surgery. I was skeptical and hesitant but I trusted the hospital's opinion." Rick smiled slightly. "I should have listened to yours instead."

"We're not against medicine," Warren said. "We just object to its stand that people are incapable of making their own choices about healthcare."

"You weren't admitted on a weekend, were you?" Ed asked cautiously.

"A Saturday morning. There was no choice, the pain was so bad."

"Not a positive indicator. Less staff working on weekends means less care."

"You think that's news," Wanda said, "Listen. You don't even know if the staff is qualified to operate. Did you read the article about the cafeteria worker who was promoted to medical assistant status because of the nurse shortage crisis?"

"Yes and that one scared me too. It's probably why other doctors are nervous about having the same surgery they perform on others, practiced on them," Ed replied.

"Hey, why don't we see if our table is ready? We can talk out there," Rick said, gesturing toward the door to the patio and Doc's well-manicured maze. "You haven't heard the best part yet."

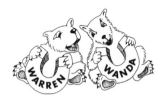

Tales of What Ails

WANDA SAT ACROSS THE TABLE FROM RICK, HER BACK TOWARD the ivy covered wall of Quackers' garden patio. "So, tell us what happened in that maze we call healthcare."

Warren sat down beside his wife. "That made you want to talk to us about it."

"Yes, we want to know," Ed said sliding into a chair beside Rick.

"My lousy habits, the ones you all mock, put me in the maze and the lousy habits the doctors and staff in there practice almost kept me in. I should have listened to you. The fact that I smoked, was overweight, didn't exercise or sleep enough, snacked all day, and worked six days a week finally caught up with me. If I'd been in better shape, my back wouldn't have deteriorated the way it did. I knew my lifestyle wasn't healthy, but I lived it anyway, and paid the price."

"You lived to work so that you could afford to live and neglected the body along the way," Ed remarked. "No wonder you ended up in the medical maze."

Rick shifted his weight in his chair to get more comfortable. "It's a maze all right. One I almost didn't escape."

"A maze full of hazards," Ed said. "When doctors in that maze don't communicate with each other and prescribe conflicting, life-threatening, drugs, some patients don't escape."

"My dear wife, Rita Linn, went crazier than our kids do at a rock concert when I was admitted. She has lost friends to medical blunders and prescription fiascos and was afraid she'd lose me. I was nervous after I read on the consent for surgical procedure form that medicine is not an exact science. I was scared when I saw that medical students were practicing on me, and how little time the over worked nurses and doctors had to care for me."

"They have to deal with a lot of pressure and mistakes are made. So what happened to you?" Ed asked.

Rick seemed hesitant. "Well, a few days after surgery my back was still sore. The nurses told me it was controlled trauma or something like that, but the next day I was in agony again. I complained, and the nurses told me it is common after surgery. I felt worse than before my surgery, though, and I was scared. I hurt and I wasn't even sure if I was going to make it."

"Hospitals are great places to go if there's no alternative," Ed said. "Let me guess: nosocomial."

"No so what?" Rick asked.

"Hospital acquired infections: the fourth most common cause of death in this country. You picked up staphylococcus aureus, a staph infection. It's a bacterium that often lives on our skin in the nose where it is harmless, but if the bacteria invade the body they can kill."

"A staph infection, yes," Rick mumbled, "at the incision site. It kept my surgical scar open. I had to stay on intravenous antibiotic treatments for weeks. My family was devastated. They knew people who died from that, too."

"Too many people," Warren said glumly. "No one's immune, especially in a hospital as overloaded as Hickory Clinic. Be thankful that you got out. This infected tissue issue of yours, this staph infection, is one of many unhealthy parts of medicine's history, one that has plagued hospitals for centuries."

"Dr. Semmelweiss, who worked at a Vienna maternity hospital in 1847, was the first to try to do something about it," Ed explained. "He made doctors wash their hands. Other doctors, proudly wearing their blood stained aprons as a status symbol, treated him like a quack for his opinions. They laughed at him for insisting that there was a link between their unwashed hands and the high mortality rate of the babies they delivered."

"Wasn't it common sense to wash your hands back then?" asked Rick.

"No, it wasn't. Doctors weren't on good terms with germs then," Warren joked. "They didn't understand how they worked."

"Even doctors today seem to have forgotten how well they work," Ed responded. "I'm dismayed at how many doctors still don't wash their hands as often as they would like you to think they do. I hear that the hospitals in England have hand-washing stations everywhere now because infections like yours are so common." Ed tucked his glasses into his shirt pocket and sighed. "That's part of the unhealthy cycle of medical history we need to put a stop to. Doctors still go from bed to bed spreading infection. According to our Center for Disease Control up the street, over two million patients die annually from the spread of germs. And that's only one example of medicine's unhealthy history that is kept filed away. Hang around, Rick, so Warren can share some more."

"How's your back doing now?" Wanda asked.

"It's still sore, but the muscle relaxants and pain medication help."

Gaia, the waitress, appeared. "Are you quacks ready to order?"

Wanda squinted slightly against the sun. "Hi, Gaia. Yeah, we're ready, but there's no hurry; we're having a long lunch today."

"I'll have the Buffalo Burger and a spinach salad, please, with the oregano farm dressing," Rick said.

Wanda put her menu back into its holder. "I'll have the Farm Raised Turkey Sandwich, with Shaman Sauce and a side of Placebo Pasta."

"And, I'll have Doc's Special please, Gaia," Warren announced, "the Body Snatcher Sandwich with the Surgeon General's Sweet and Sour Sauce."

Ed thought a moment. "Let me have your soup of the day, the Witches' Gruel, and the Soy and Goat Cheese Melt sandwich with spelt bread, please."

"On its healthy way," Gaia said cheerfully, flipping the page of her order pad over and heading toward the next table.

"So, tell me, why does Doc use all these crazy names on his menu?" Rick asked.

"Like AMA for Alternative Meat Appetizers or FDA for Food, Drinks, and Aperitifs? Because it keeps customers amused," Wanda said. "And Doc likes to stir things up. He put 'Don't Panic, Eat Organic' on the menu in response to the concerns about genetically modified foods and he planted a real maze in the garden area behind you as a protest against the maze medicine had become. A maze you got caught in, and moved through, my friend; moved," Wanda repeated, "like a magnet."

"Moved like a magnet?" Rick said.

"It's a metaphor," Wanda said playing with her hair. "We've teased you before about being moved like a magnet through the medical maze. How positive health habits keep you out of it and negative habits pull you into it. If you are moving your own magnet, it means that you've taken responsibility for your own health and can't be moved like how a magnet is moved, by a force stronger than itself, through the medical maze."

"It's a loose metaphor, Rick," Warren explained. "The emphasis isn't on which poles attract and which repel, but on the influence medicine and the food and drug industries have on your health."

"And how little influence you have on it yourself," Ed added.

"So, if I take responsibility for my health and walk the middle path to wellness - the self-care instead of the managed care path - I influence how my health is managed and move my own magnet?"

Wanda eagerly agreed, "That's right. Unhealthy people with negative habits who don't take responsibility for their healthcare get drawn like the weak magnets they represent, into the health-care maze. Healthy people see the medical maze for what it is and only enter the maze for supportive solutions like stitches or setting bones. They might use medical technology for a diagnosis but they will always explore natural treatments first."

Rick leaned back and rested both hands on his protruding belly. "So, I'm a weak magnet drawn to medicine because of my sorry health habits and by what I believe medicine can, and must, do for me."

"By changing your lifestyle, you can become a strong magnet," Ed suggested.

"Ah, change," Rick said, rolling his thumbs around each other. "Now that's something to wrestle with isn't it? Hickory Clinic gave me a jolt, but was it a big enough one to make me want to change my ways? I'm not sure."

"Only you can decide to take responsibility for your health, Rick, and move your own magnet," Wanda replied. "But, by accepting responsibility for yourself you also set an example for others to follow."

"And become a Wellness Wombat," Ed said.

Rick looked confused. "A Wellness Wombat; what's that?"

"I know you love kids, Rick. Well, the Wellness Wombats were born while I was telling mine a bedtime story," Warren replied happy to be telling his story again. "A bus full of tourists, on their way to Sydney stopped by the road to take a junk food break and left their trash behind; wombats ate from it, got sick and swore they'd never let their kids make the same mistake. A wombat is a cuddly koala bear-like Australian animal that lives in a burrow, or warren. A Wellness Wombat is anyone who is health conscious and who by word of mouth shares with others how they can become healthy, too."

"Anyone who lives the same way we do, basically," Wanda confirmed. "Anyone who eats right and stays away from fast foods, lives in harmony with nature, and seeks out natural alternative remedies over synthetic or medical ones, and sees the medical maze as a last resort instead of the first stop. WOMBAT is an acronym, Rick; it stands for word of mouth business all the time, something everyone is in whether they realize it or not."

"Well, your Wellness Wombats certainly make being healthy sound like fun. The kids I teach at church would like the idea." Rick hesitated. "And, if it will keep me out of the medical maze, I might even be open to it. Except, I'm not sure where I would start."

Wanda spoke first. "Begin by reading life's labels, Rick, the signs that nature and your own body give you, instead of the ones you find on prescriptions or packaged food."

"That's right. Take it one step at a time," Warren said, happy to debate the point. "Buy organic. Cook at home. Reduce and replace. Reduce the salt. Replace it with herbs. Reduce the saturated fats. Replace them with olive oil.

Reduce the soda. Replace it with water. Reduce the sugar. Replace it with stevia. You get the picture."

"Keep it simple," Wanda said. "Start with herbs, organic fruits and vegetables, clean water, fresh air, exercise, and plenty of sleep. You know, the basic stuff."

"It sounds so simple, so obvious," Rick said, patting his belly, "but it's hard to do."

"You just have to be willing," Wanda said, "like so many of my Charter Spa members were when I first opened." She paused to smile. "At first, you'll wrestle with the new habits a healthy lifestyle requires, but they'll become second nature eventually. Besides, you'll feel so good practicing these new habits that you won't want to go back to feeling the way you did before."

Warren pulled out his wallet and placed a laminated card with red text on the table. "Here's a checklist I created," he said, staring at Rick, "It might help you answer the where do I start question that you asked earlier."

Rick read the title: "Five Ways to Stay Out of the Maze."

"The Five Elements of Chinese Medicine inspired this card," Warren said. "They'll help you manage your health and move your own magnet, instead of being drawn like one into the maze we call medicine. Go ahead. Read them if you want."

"Number one: Be conscious of what you are fed by the world, by food and drug companies, by medicine, and by the media messiahs. Don't get drawn into their ways.

Number two: Respect your body and help it help itself by giving it the time and environment it needs every day to get regular exercise, proper nutrition, clean water, clean air, and sufficient sleep.

Hmm," Rick muttered, "every day, huh?" He held the laminated card at an angle to counteract the light reflecting off it, and squinted briefly.

"Number three: Go outside. Nurture your connection to nature. Listen to the rhythm and pulse of your body, and your intuition. It will tell you what is good for you.

"What's this mean?" Rick asked.

Wanda explained. "Health by intuition I call it. And most city dwellers have lost touch with their intuition. It means the better you treat your body, physically and emotionally, the more you are in rhythm with its natural pulse and the pulse of nature. And the more it is in rhythm with you. Then you can intuitively know when you no longer need things like sugar, caffeine, alcohol, or tobacco. We know a lot of people who do this. It keeps them healthy and out of the medical maze."

"So, it's not too late for me, then?" Rick said with a grin, looking at the card again.

"Number four: Address stress. Spend more time being still and less time being busy."

"Busy being what and where others expect you to be, that is," Wanda explained.

"That's way out there," Rick said rubbing his back briefly. "How does anybody find time to just be still?"

"Most don't," Warren replied, "that's why they're so stressed out and never get to number two on the card you're reading."

"Instead of working overtime, try working 'over time.' Spread out your work and don't stress over it," Ed calmly suggested. "Today's number one killer is stress. Nearly every doctor I work with at Hickory Clinic will tell you that. Try and design your life with less stress. Try yoga or meditation, or just get away from your work space and find a quiet place to take time out."

"I'm game, if it will keep me out of the medical maze," Rick replied. "Okay, let me see."

"Number five: Walk the middle path to wellness; don't depend on alternative or traditional care. Self-care is better for you than the maze we call healthcare."

"The middle path I talked about earlier," Warren confirmed. "It's easier to stay on it if you heed number one on this list. In fact, you can practice being conscious of what you are fed right here at Quackers."

"Ah, but it's not just about eating Doc's organic food," Ed cautioned. "It's also about how you eat it. I work with a lot of dieticians at the hospital and here's something they taught me: masticate now and you won't have to medicate later. Salivary glands and natural digestive enzymes in the stomach break down a meal; if you have a drink with a meal their capacity to do that is diluted and you end up taking antacids because the food is coming up instead of breaking down. So, check in with your stomach before you put more food into your mouth. You don't have to eat those giant portions that restaurants serve today, especially if you're already full. You've got to eat slowly, too: chew your food. Respect the effort it took to bring it to the table. Respect how it serves your body. Don't make eating a stressful experience."

"And treat eating like an inconvenience, you mean?" Rick said.

"That's right," Ed replied. "The ugly secret behind the success of convenience food is this: they have convinced us that eating, and especially cooking, is inconvenient. But there's nothing convenient about the health it takes away from you later. So, respect the body that serves you by serving it better fuel, or prescription drugs will fuel you later."

Rick ran his fingers along the edge of the laminated card. "I like your checklist, Warren, but I just don't know how I'm going to apply it, especially after being conditioned to ignore it for so long by the conveniences that Main Street and medicine have sold me on over the years," Rick continued. "Look, I know you're trying to give me a map out of the medical maze, here, and save me from my unhealthy ways. But as scared as I am of medicine now, I can't just jump into this alternative stuff. Besides, negative health habits are part of my nature by now.

I'm the unhealthy lifestyle guy remember? My hospital experience changed my views, but I can't guarantee it will change my habits. Anyway, like I said, I've got to take care of me right now. And the only way I know to do that is to get back to work as soon as I can to support my family, which means these five ways out of the maze are going to have to wait a while. It sounds hypocritical, I know, but there it is."

Wanda spoke up again. "We understand. You came to us for advice; you have to choose how you use it."

Rick put the laminated card down on the table and smiled. "Hey, I know you want to help, but your way of thinking about your health is different from mine. Our lifestyles are poles apart."

Wanda returned the smile. "We are trying to help you change that thinking, Rick, that's all. We consider you a friend and we care about you. We can't help you if you don't want help. It's been fun ribbing each other about our different lifestyles, but you're on the other side of the fence now. Your unhealthy habits put you into the hospital. They'll put you in there again if you don't change them."

"Relax, Rick. Enjoy your lunch and listen to what the Wellness Wombats have to say," Warren pleaded. "I think you'll find it fun hearing their stories about ways to stay out of the maze."

Wanda deliberately stared at Rick's large belly. "You survived Hickory Clinic this time, but if you go back to your unhealthy ways you'll be the weak magnet again and you'll get moved like one right back into that medical maze."

"She's right," Ed said, taking his glasses out of his pocket and putting them back on. "Take it from a doctor. Medicine has become as sick as the people it treats. You might come out of its maze in a coffin next time."

"We understand your resistance, Rick," Warren said, putting both elbows on the table. "Adopting a healthy lifestyle takes years. We don't expect you to drop your burger binge-ing, soda sucking, pizza poking, T.V. toting lifestyle overnight. But we do expect to help you change it. You did ask us for help, didn't you?"

Rick sighed. "Yeah, I did. But, I'm just wrestling with the changes you're proposing, even though I want to defy the doctors' predictions and avoid further back surgery."

Warren reached for the card Rick had been reading, picked it up and looked at Rick. "Here, take this home," he instructed. "Stick it on the fridge or something; at least try number one."

"My wife will think I've been around you folks too long if I stick this on my fridge."

Ed gave Rick a friendly nudge. "Tell her you're determined to beat the statistics and live longer than she will. Tell her that your friends at Quackers have invited you to become a Wellness Wombat. If Warren makes them a reality, that is."

Rick picked up the card and looked at Warren. "And just when do you think I'm going to find time to practice these five ways to stay out of the maze?"

"Please make time, Rick," Warren begged. "If you don't, you might have less time on this planet and we want you to stick around. We want you well, so you can pass on what we taught you to your kids, and they can by word of mouth pass it on too. Just imagine how many people we can keep out of the medical maze then."

"You want me to become a Wellness Wombat, in other words."

"We don't want you to be a wombat in combat who has to storm the walls of the medical maze," Warren said persuasively. "That's a job reserved for a committed advocate like me, who gets up early to battle bills at The State Capitol that cement the power medicine has over how you manage your health. We don't want you to change the way medicine operates; we want you to change the way you operate. We want you to get well and stay well. The more people like you who do that, the more medicine will see how quickly they must change the ways of their maze."

Rick slid the card into his pocket. "Getting on the alternative path is a big step. I know I've got to change my ways, and move my own magnet, as you put it, but I have a hard time passing by a donut shop without buying something. I'd make a pretty sorry Wellness Wombat."

Warren leaned closer to Rick and looked him in the eye again. "Let me ask you a question. Medicine always asks you about your history, doesn't it?"

"You mean my medical history?" Rick asked.

"Yes, your medical history. Did you ever bother to ask about medicine's history?"

Rick was caught off guard. "Er, no," he said. "I just took it for granted that doctors knew what they were doing."

"My point exactly," Warren declared, leaning back in his chair and tapping his hand on the table. "Why don't we take a look at its history? It's not as healthy as you think."

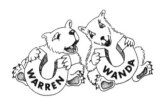

An Impatient History

"I'M NOT AS HEALTHY AS I THOUGHT I WAS; THAT'S WHY I'M here," Rick reminded everyone.

"And why you ended up over there." Warren gestured toward Hickory Clinic and then drummed his hands on the table again. "I think it's time to let my Wellness Wombat characters walk you through medicine's history, Rick. Then you'll see how the maze you got caught in convinced you it was your only alternative."

"The characters he's talking about are the wellness advocates who fought for the right to choose how they managed their health centuries ago," Wanda quickly explained.

"I know," Rick said, "and used the word of mouth business to do it. That's where the WOMBAT acronym came from."

"This is the fun version of the message we kept repeating before you went into the hospital," Warren said, obviously enjoying his audience. "That once you discover the truth behind how hard medicine works to keep you in its maze, you'll want to work harder at keeping yourself healthy.

Something more internet savvy consumers are doing: becoming better informed so they won't have to be at the mercy of medicine. They're demanding the alternatives that medicine has kept from them, too."

"Medicine has suppressed alternative care for centuries because it's threatened," Doctor Ed remarked. "Today the American Medical Association and the local medical boards want to forcibly integrate those alternatives. That way, they can be the ones who dictate how they are practiced."

"Which brings us full circle to the suppressive tactics medicine used centuries ago to direct people away from alternatives in the first place," Wanda said, "tactics Warren's Wellness Wombats reveal in his ten stage history."

"A history I'm keen to hear," Ed said. "Let's get started."

Warren took a deep breath. "Okay. I should start by quoting a favorite Wellness Wombat of mine, Doctor Benjamin Rush, founding father of American Medicine and signer of The Declaration of Independence. He said: "If medical freedom were not put into the Constitution, then medicine would organize itself into an undercover dictatorship." Doctor Rush foresaw how consuming the medical trap would become, as did generations of Wellness Wombats before and after him." Warren turned toward Rick. "Do you remember the story I told you about the wombats that got sick from the junk food tourists left on the side of the road?"

"I do," Rick replied. "They helped other wombats avoid the same mistake by teaching them to stick to the diet nature had provided."

"Well, from that little tale the Wellness Wombats were born. So were the stories I'm going to share with you about witches, gravediggers, body snatchers, and bloodletters. Stories about wellness advocates who, through every stage of medicine's unhealthy history, fought to keep alternative medicine alive. Now these stories aren't in any particular timeline. I jump around a bit because I want to alert you to how the medical maze was built, not give you a chronological history of medicine."

Rick grinned. "Go ahead; I'm all ears."

Warren took a deep breath. "I've called Stage One: The Witch and the Woodcutter. It's about the hoax medicine played that wrestled away the rights of the people to heal themselves, and the power plays upon which the foundations of the medical maze were built."

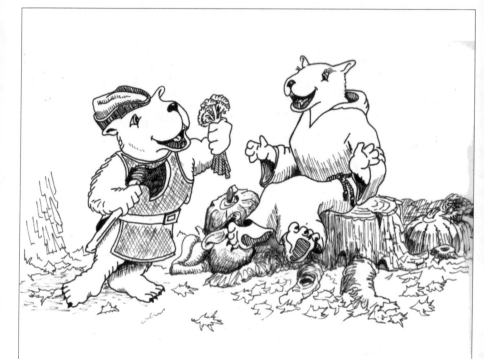

When Godfrey cut wood, he collected plants and herbs that Gwen used to treat people in the village.

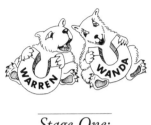

Stage One:

The Witch and the Woodcutter

"So," Rick asked curiously, "Is the woodcutter our first Wellness Wombat?"

"Yes," Warren replied in his storyteller voice. "Godfrey, a fourteenth century woodsman, was a Wellness Wombat because he loved nature. His friend Gwen, the natural healer or, witch, as she was later branded, loved nature, too. When Godfrey cut wood he collected plants and herbs that Gwen used to treat people in the village. Gwen could cure just about anything and her knowledge of the healing powers of herbs and plants threatened those in authority who claimed that her apparent skills were not based on the scientific facts of the day but on superstition, folklore, and hearsay."

"So they branded her as a witch and burned her at the stake?" Rick asked.

"They did indeed. In medieval Europe men held positions of power, but one power they didn't have was the power to heal. Women held that power. Men were threatened by that power, just as medicine is today. Men of the church, mostly, who controlled the souls of their followers through fear: the fear that their souls wouldn't go to heaven if they committed whatever the church decided at the moment was a sin.

"They couldn't control our woodsman friend, our medieval Wellness Wombat. He and his friends knew how to heal themselves. Or which witch to go to. They had no fear. Neither did the church leaders, for they branded all villagers who followed the old ways of healing as troublemakers and ridiculed them as sinners who were performing the devil's work. They accused healers of being evil as well, and branded those as witches who practiced dangerous black magic, not healers providing proven natural remedies. Of course, the church felt that it was their job to protect the villagers from evil so they got away with accusing healers of practicing witchcraft, consorting with the devil, and even got away with burning them."

"Condemning them to the stake, you mean," Wanda declared.

"That's right. Godfrey had noticed an increased demand for wood. He had seen local magistrates grabbing unsuspecting villagers, mostly women, and jabbing them with a device that pricked their skin. If it didn't make the victim bleed, the magistrate publicly accused the woman of being a witch and hauled her off to be condemned."

"Talk about getting caught in the medical trap," Ed said with a grin.

"Prickers, as they were called, trapped a lot of people, Ed. They secretly fixed their device to retract so it wouldn't break the skin. If someone didn't bleed, she wasn't considered human, and was immediately accused of consorting with evil. Fear of sin was so great that church leaders, jealous rivals, and local magistrates had no problem bribing prickers to dispose of innocent troublemakers."

"So, let me guess," Rick said, piecing the information

together. "Our Wellness Wombat rushed back to the village to warn his healer friend, the witch."

"That's right. And when he got there she was already tied to the stake. Godfrey stumbled into the center of the village and was horrified to see his wood and Gwen, his witch friend, burning at the same time. Sorry to say, the villagers just stood around and watched. I guess when you've got the power of the church putting the fear of God's wrath and the threat of torture into you, watching someone else burn for practicing black magic is easier than condemning yourself to the same fire."

Wanda looked puzzled. "America had its share of witch hunting, didn't it Warren?"

"Yes. Thirty years after England outlawed the practice, America was still burning witches: Salem in 1692; New York City in 1741; and, in 1770, somewhere in Illinois, two more witches were burned. I think the monarchy and the church burned witches to convince people that local troublemakers were the cause of their problems, not those who ruled over and taxed them. But the truth is that the clergy, magistrates, and lords wanted any quacks practicing medicine in their territory to be practicing it in a way that they could control. They wanted their version of medicine practiced not some alternative to it. This is the original hoax, Rick. Those in power took away the powers and the rights of the people to heal themselves."

"The first stage of the disease we call medicine," Wanda suggested. "Medicine ridiculed what people had always practiced by calling it superstition. It wrestled traditions away, then re-labeled them as traditional medicine and practiced them anyway."

"The hoax, or practice, now known as conventional or, traditional, medicine," Doctor Ed said, "is the foundation on which today's medical maze is built."

Rick looked worried. "So, what did our woodcutter do? Did he fight back?"

"Godfrey did the only thing he could do, Rick. He became a wellness advocate. Yes, a Wellness Wombat. And he fought back by passing on, by word of mouth, the knowledge healers who were being burned at the stake had used. In his own quiet way he took a stand for nature's ways and spoke up whenever he could, against the ways of the maze. A role wellness advocates have had to play ever since," Warren said.

Rick shook his head as though coming out of a dream. "You make it sound so real."

"It is real, very real," Warren concluded. "And if the Bills I'm fighting at The State Capitol that restrict people's rights to choose how they manage their health pass, then what happened to our woodcutter and witch will happen to us. The wellness movement we are seeing today can break this pattern if it wants to, before it infects another generation by taking away its rights to freely purchase alternative remedies and supplements without a doctor's prescription."

"So, you're telling me that your alternative medicine was once mainstream traditional medicine?" Rick asked.

"Yes! This is what Dr. Benjamin Rush was warning us about. This is the hoax that set out to wrestle away the rights our Wellness Wombat woodsman had to pursue his own self-care and force him to submit to traditional medicine's healthcare instead. This hoax needs to be revealed exactly for what it is, so that people will stop to think before they just automatically follow their doctors' orders to swallow each and every pill they prescribe. We, the people, simply cannot turn over all responsibility for our own well-being and the right to heal ourselves to medicine or to our elected officials.

"Don't paint too dark a picture," Wanda commented thoughtfully. "Medicine infects the public with its negatives, but it has its positives, too. Alternative medicine has its quacks, but there are quacks in traditional medicine too, like the physicians who hide patient records to avoid malpractice suits."

"You have to be as wary today of a doctor who believes in everything medicine promotes, just as you would have had to a hundred years ago," Doctor Ed said. "But, I give my colleagues at Hickory Clinic a pat on the back. I see more of them recommending massage, exercise, diet, even yoga and meditation, these days."

Warren leaned forward. "Perhaps when they hear these stories about the history behind the construction of the medical maze, they'll have a bigger incentive to recommend alternatives and encourage people to stay out of that maze by questioning a healthcare model that insists on connecting you with a medical doctor every time you feel sick.

"If people would just stop to ask themselves a few questions before religiously marching into emergency rooms and taking whatever the doctor recommends, this country wouldn't be in the healthcare mess it's in."

Rick looked puzzled. "What kind of questions?"

Warren spoke firmly but slowly. "Like, am I attracted to or repelled by this aspect of healthcare? Is it moving my magnet for me or is it helping me to move my own? Does it support or repress my rights? Help or hinder how I manage my own health?"

Rick sipped his juice. "Good questions. So, witches: sorry, I mean women, influenced the first stage of the construction of the medical maze. What happened next?"

"The hoax that the men in power played to secure their position and suffocate people's rights to heal themselves was stage one. They dealt women a breath-robbing blow by wrestling their healing powers and practices away from them in order to construct their medical maze. Now they had to expand upon the territory claimed from that match. They had to establish territory or, turf, on which they could practice and profit from the right to heal that they were trying to secure."

"We're still in the fourteenth century, right?" Wanda inquired.

"Yes," Warren replied. "We're talking about claiming and guarding territory or turf now, territory to practice in and territory to protect the profits that practice produced."

"That sounds like the way medicine is practiced in this century," Ed said.

Warren had an answer. "It's the cycle of medical history I talk about all the time. Medicine is defeated if its sick practices aren't repeated."

"Hmm," Ed said, "I'll have to remember that one."

"Remember, back then both sides referred to the other as quacks," Warren stressed. "Practitioners of new medicine and natural medicine were both suspicious of each other. For centuries, new medicine had been working hard to convince people to trust it, and in the end it won out. It conditioned people to view alternative natural medicine as quackery and secured the ground it needed on which to build its medical maze. Meanwhile, people like Godfrey, who were willing to take responsibility for their health, and rely on nature's ways to do it, had to be on their guard and stay out of the maze."

"In case they got branded as a witch, you mean?"

"Yes, Rick," Warren said seriously, "like natural therapists who get branded today, sometimes even jailed, for promoting natural cures for cancer and other diseases that medicine claims only it can cure. Anyway, you won't be surprised if I tell you that my next story is about a guard at the local castle. Our wood cutting Wellness Wombat sold wood there."

Rick winced slightly from the pain in his back as he shifted his weight in his chair. "So, were they buddies?" He asked.

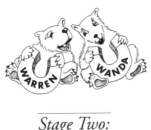

Stage Two:

The Guard at the Gate and the Cook Who Couldn't Wait

WARREN SET THE STAGE. "MEL, THE GUARD, WAS AN OLD friend of Godfrey's from the same village. Mel believed in nature's remedies and the old ways too. But, while being a guard Mel, like Godfrey, had to be on guard, and keep quiet about any natural cures or remedies he used. The Lord of the castle whose territory he protected used fear to stay in power.

The use of fear helped the hoax practitioners of new medicine were playing work. Fear forced the villagers into believing that the old medicine, the natural medicine so-called witches practiced, was unproven, unsafe and, now, unauthorized. Medicine used fear tactics to convince castle dwellers and local common folk that the new medicine, even though it was the old medicine re-labeled, was not quackery, and that the doctors practicing it were not quacks."

"Early medicine had the same fight on its hands then as it does today," Ed commented, "that of convincing people the ways of the maze aren't questionable quackery."

"Early medicine had other battles to fight, too. Feudal lords like the one Godfrey worked for could execute doctors

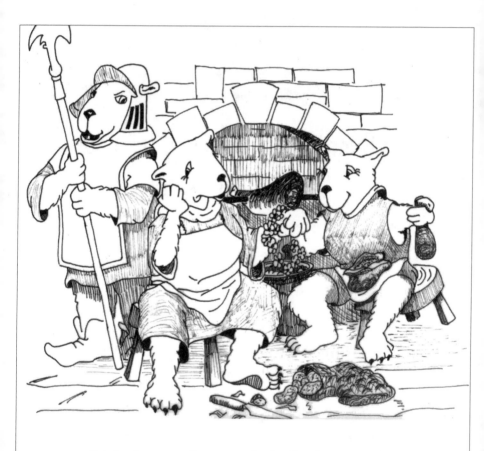

Mel, the guard, smuggled a healer into the
castle kitchen. The healer tied violets around
the cooks' wrist to check her fever.

for killing patients: for malpractice," Warren recalled. "But, back to my story. The castle that Mel guarded welcomed important guests: the magistrates, the clergy, and practitioners of the new medicine. It even welcomed the prickers who had condemned Godfrey's friend Gwen to death. The practitioners of the new medicine practiced their craft on their benefactors, the men in power, and on the villagers who worked at the castle. Of course, they blamed anything that didn't work on witchcraft in order to avoid the quack label Mel the guard and his Wellness Wombat friends gave them."

Ed smiled. "Practitioners of new medicine were eager to set up a practice, to establish a reputation and a territory."

"So did they get to practice on Mel, the guard?" Wanda asked. "Our Wellness Wombat?"

"No way, but they almost got the guard's friend, Matilda the cook. This story is about both of them, the guard at the gate and the cook who couldn't wait. You see, when our chubby guard, Mel, wasn't at the gatehouse guarding the entrance to the castle or in the kitchen getting fed extra scraps by Matilda the cook, he was watching the new men of medicine wander around the castle to experiment on servants, soldiers, and stable lads.

Mel quickly figured out that the quackery he had learned from Gwen the witch who had been burned at the stake for practicing it, was safer than the new medicine they were practicing. Mel knew he'd better be on his guard if he wanted to avoid new medicine's territory. His guard, and his allegiance to the so-called quackery he trusted, was soon put to the test."

"Let me guess," Wanda said. "The cook got sick and was about to become the next guinea pig for your new healers to practice on."

Warren grinned, pleased with his audience's participation. "You got it! Now Mel had to decide: will he risk helping his friend with remedies that he favors, the old medicine, or will he subject Matilda to the ways of the maze, the new medicine?"

"If he was ruled by fear he would submit to the hoax even though he didn't believe in it," Rick answered. "He would put the cook in the new healer's hands. If he was caught practicing that alternative stuff, he'd be persecuted, or even prosecuted."

"Which is why he has to be on his guard," Warren responded, still grinning. "But Matilda couldn't wait to get away from the hands of the new practitioners and into the hands of someone she trusted. She asked Mel, the guard, to send a message to the woodcutter to find a natural healer. Mel smuggled one past the marshals, bailiffs, and other watchmen, into the depths of the castle kitchen. The healer tied violets around the cook's wrist to check her fever. The quicker they wither, the higher the fever. Then she administered horehound for her cough, mullein leaf tea to soothe her inflamed throat, the herb boneset to induce sweating, and caraway root to chew on. The cook got well."

Warren looked directly at Rick again. "So, Mel became our Wellness Wombat because he not only protected and guarded others from falling prey to the new ways if they got sick, but he guarded the old ways too. He passed them on, or made sure they got passed on. He also displayed the same mistrust of medicine that people have today. And Mel, along with Godfrey, and their Wellness Wombat friends, did something about medicine's ill ways. They used the power of word of mouth to discredit it. They didn't let the new medicine's practitioners mock, suppress, or replace the old ways. They made sure everyone knew that quackery was very much alive in both fields of medicine."

"Which is what you are hoping your modern day Wellness Wombats will do, right? If you can attract enough of them and make everyone aware that there are quacks everywhere, both in alternative and traditional medicine?"

"Right again, Rick, but I don't want people who become Wellness Wombats to set out to discredit medicine, or even tout alternative medicine as the only answer. I want them to be leery, like the guard and the cook, of how they are steered away from nature's ways, and led instead into the medical maze."

Ed jumped in. "More people are leery today. They come into doctor's offices, like mine, better informed than they used to be and question our methods and motives. They often choose alternative treatments before opting for traditional ones. They are becoming Wellness Wombats without even knowing it."

"I wish I'd chosen alternatives, knowing what I know now," Rick admitted.

"Hickory Clinic opened your eyes, didn't it?" Ed said. "Don't worry Warren's going to open them even wider. He should have already with his first two stories. Scary, isn't it, that doctors have been 'practicing' medicine for centuries. Even scarier that they managed to bury the hoax they pulled off when they wrestled medicine away from witch-healers too."

"About as scary as the consent form I signed before going into surgery. The one that says medicine is not an exact science," Rick agreed. "I thought they knew what they were doing. Give them some credit though, they did manage to turn the medicine they wrestled away, and the 'quack' reputations they had for how they interpreted it into something stable enough to gain the peoples' trust."

"A trust secured by intimidation," Doctor Ed said. "The physical intimidation the prickers practiced has turned into the psychological intimidation that doctors use today when they imply that their ways, not the old ways, are better, and that technology heals, not nature."

"Medicine became pretty good at minimizing the validity of alternative, natural medicine in the next few stages of its history." Warren said. "This stage of the maze's construction is about its quest to secure trust and shake off its own quack label. It's about medicine's quest to establish itself and its territory so that it would be seen as the one with the power to heal."

"Let me guess," Rick interjected, "by promoting the medical maze, not nature's ways."

"To attract people, like a magnet, into that maze," Wanda added, "a maze that more people are repelled by these days."

"Repelled because of the efforts of people like our woodcutter and castle guard who strove to keep alternative remedies alive and who, by word of mouth, passed their benefits on. Modern day Wellness Wombats don't want the ways of the maze to dominate public health anymore either; they want the right to freely choose who manages their health."

"I have a question," Rick said. "Did doctors, in their eagerness to secure turf, and establish territory, which is what you are telling me this stage of the maze's construction is about, get the support they needed from those in power?"

"No," Warren answered, "they didn't. Sometimes those in power were Wellness Wombats. At least when it pleased them, they were. Henry VIII is famous for burning the monasteries down in 1536, and for having many wives, but he's not so well known for being the first to pass anti-witchcraft laws and seeking to control the authority that the doctors wanted for themselves. The Quacks Charter that he passed in 1542, which Doc fixed to Quackers front door when he first opened for business, talks about that."

"I haven't read what's on the front door in a while; remind me," Rick said.

"Doctors from prestigious universities wanted their competition, that is, anyone who practiced natural medicine, the uneducated 'pagan' healers as they were so called, kept at bay. They asked the King to restrict unlicensed practitioners from operating on their turf. That's what really happened. But Henry VIII was an advocate of herbal remedies and wanted the poor to have access to them. He knew the poor couldn't afford doctors, and he also knew his treasury couldn't afford to support them. So, he passed the Quacks Charter in 1542 and made it legal for herbalists to heal people with their medicines, too."

"Medicine still protects its turf or, territory, today," Ed sighed, "by prescribing synthetic drugs over herbal remedies. It's the cycle of medical history in gear again, the repetitive pattern you referred to Warren: a pattern that will only change when doctors take alternative medicine more seriously and traditional medicine less seriously."

"Okay," Rick said, patting his belly fondly, "let me get clear about the message in the stories about your Wellness Wombats because you make it all sound so obvious. Men used to having power, or taking it, went from Stage One: the wrestling away of the ability to heal, to Stage Two: establishing territory or, turf, on which they could practice and profit from the right they had secured to heal."

"You got it, and this is the pattern medicine recycles throughout its unhealthy history in order to strengthen or defend its maze," Warren said. "It's the condition that's plagued us for centuries, and forced both fields of medicine to battle the other for position and fight to gain the trust of a public that simply wants to stay well. Anyway, on to Stage Three: the plagues. And to my next Wellness Wombat story, about a gravedigger who survived the plague."

"Oh, good," Rick said, "death and destruction, my favorite part of history. Now it's getting interesting."

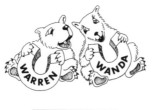

Stage Three:

Garlic for the Gravedigger

"THE BLACK DEATH THAT HIT LONDON IN 1348 IS WHAT'S interesting," Warren began, setting the tone for his next tale. "London had grown too fast and its streets were full of rotting garbage, human waste, and flea-ridden, plague carrying rats. It's the ideal setting for my next story, which I've called: Garlic for the Gravedigger. But, before I tell the story, let me share a little background.

"You see, cities like London hadn't always been so unsanitary. In the fifth century, before the plagues spread across Europe and killed one-third of the population, the Roman Empire ruled. The Romans had strict rules about sanitation and personal hygiene and brought order, hygiene, education, and commerce to any territory they conquered."

"I read somewhere that Romans were not big on doctors or medicine because their high sanitary standards limited the need for them," Ed said.

"True," Warren replied. "They created those disease-defying standards by using the slave labor of the armies they defeated

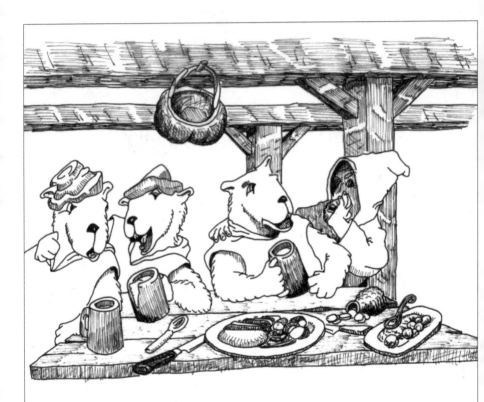

A mysterious character walked into the tavern
and whispered into Mort's ear.

to build leak-resistant aqueducts that fed clean running water into their baths, spas, and sewage systems. But, sadly, the Roman Empire crumbled and their sanitary practices were lost. Centuries later, disease ruled instead. By the time we reach the fourteenth century, disease had spread across Europe. France and Italy were the first to quarantine and contain it. Both avoided the full force of the plague when they shut city gates to keep residents in and travelers out and then quarantined merchant ships. London, however, wasn't so smart. The Great Plague hit it hard."

"You told me that this was the stage in the construction of the medical maze when Public Health Boards were born. Am I right?" Wanda inquired.

"You're right. But let me tell you the story about our gravedigger Wellness Wombat, then you will know why." Warren lowered his voice. "You see, Mort, our gravedigger, was a wise and friendly old shepherd from the country where the only remedies he relied on if he got sick were nature-based." Warren spoke a little faster. "Today we would call him a health nut. It was the year 1348 and Mort had come to London in search of work a week before the Great Plague. He got a job as a gravedigger; a job that kept him knee-deep in graves, trampling over stiff, bloated corpses every day."

"How did he survive that?" Rick asked.

"He was very healthy because he had lived in the country-side," Warren answered. "He had a strong immune system. He also had a secret remedy to keep the plague at bay. He drank a lot of beer and mulled red wine."

"What's mulled red wine?"

"Good question, Rick. It was a popular medieval drink packed with herbs, spices, and cloves, and served warm. Our gravedigger drank lots of it with his green cheese and boiled bacon lunch. He chewed on eryngo root, too, a gum-like substance well known for guarding against infections back then, but his real secret was the raw wild white garlic he ate every day. This natural antidote protected him so that he could bury people all day long without fear of getting the plague.

"One day, a mysterious character wearing a dark cloak walked uncertainly into the tavern, approached our Wellness Wombat, and whispered into his ear. "My master is a powerful leader of the church and has heard of your ability to avoid the plague. He will pay you for this knowledge. He does not trust his medical practitioners. They want to bleed him, read his urine and his planets, check the color of his bile, and sit him in front of fires to sweat. Will you help him survive the plague and share your secret?

"Our wise old Wellness Wombat laughed at first, because the clergy had mocked his friends' superstitious ways and cruelly set out to replace them with their own quackery. Now they wanted to protect themselves from the plague by using remedies that they had once scorned and discouraged."

"Did our Wellness Wombat take the money he was offered?" Rick asked.

"He took it on the condition that his remedy be shared. He wanted the lessons the priests learned on how to get well passed on into the community and made public. He wanted alternative, preventative, practices, the old ways, not just the ways of the maze kept alive. Now to Wanda's question; the success of the quarantining policy that France and Italy began served as a great example of early public health management. In the post plague of the thirteen fifties it also led to the creation, by most European cities, of Boards of Public Health. To avoid future plagues, leaders realized Public Health Boards should be set up to enforce sanitary standards and take responsibility for the health of their city."

"Something the Romans had learned centuries ago, right?" Rick said.

"That's right," Warren replied. "Now listen to this, because there's another hoax buried in the files of medicine's history in this stage. Ed reminded us about the lack of respect the Romans had for medicine. They didn't trust doctors. Well, these first Public Health Boards didn't, either. They wanted to protect the public from future plagues by setting sanitary standards. They wanted to protect the public from medicine, too. They promptly shut down doctors and potion-carrying quacks, no matter how well the remedies they peddled worked. Even the Pope's practitioners couldn't practice their quackery anymore."

"By shutting down quacks, the Public Health Boards opened the door for the public to move their own magnet again, didn't they?" Ed asked. "They mimicked the Romans by practicing common sense health and hygiene habits, and walked the middle path by not relying on quacks in either field of medicine, but were responsible for their own health."

"Yes. After the plague, public morale and health were low, and distrust of quacks in both fields of medicine, and the church - which hadn't protected body or soul during the plague - was high. But the plague's devastation had led to another realization: how little doctors, or anyone in authority really knew, and how much quackery was practiced in both fields of medicine."

"Enter the medical schools!" Ed announced.

"Enter the medical schools," Warren echoed, turning to Rick. "This is the stage that spawned Public Health Boards and medical schools, Rick. Both expanded their influence. It's an important phase in the construction of the maze."

Rick scratched his head. "There weren't any medical schools before the Great Plague?"

"Or any plagues before The Great Plague?" Warren teased. "There were both, of course. The Justinian Plague in Constantinople in 452AD and a medical school in Salerno, Italy, in the ninth century. But our point is that Public Health Boards didn't just impose new sanitary standards. They wanted medical practitioners to meet those standards, too. So, they encouraged medical schools to open and provide certified doctors who knew what they were doing."

"In the fifteenth century there were schools in Bologna, Paris, and Oxford," Ed said with a chuckle, "and I think they did what they knew; though they didn't necessarily know what they were doing."

"The early medical schools thought they had the panacea, the 'cure-all.' They taught their medical students to demote natural healers and their potions, and promote doctors and their lotions instead. This leads me into Stage Four, a short story this time, about the herb lady's potions and the doctor's lotions. My next character is Heather the herb lady. Her busy stall was part of a market outside the grounds of a fifteenth century London medical school."

"At last, a woman," Wanda sighed.

"Yes. In fact, a woman very much like you," Warren said with a warm smile.

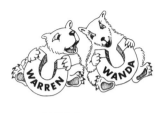

Stage Four:

The Herb Lady's Potions and the Doctor's Lotions

"HEATHER THE HERB LADY BELIEVED IN WHAT SHE HAD SEEN work and questioned the practices so-called doctors were promoting. Practices the public saw as quackery." Warren looked back at Rick. "Anyway, this story reveals yet another phase of the creation of the medical maze. It spotlights a doctrine that cemented the maze's construction that medical schools taught then, and still pass down today; one that launched a few too many ego-driven doctors along the way. The doctrine was founded on how impressed medicine was by itself and its discoveries and went like this: the human body is far too complex for people to heal; only medicine can manage the public's health now."

"So, what people fell for then, we're still falling for today," Rick said.

"The Public Health Boards didn't fall for it right away. Eventually medicine had to back their cure-all claims with scientific studies, but it's a doctrine that has plagued medicine and the public for centuries."

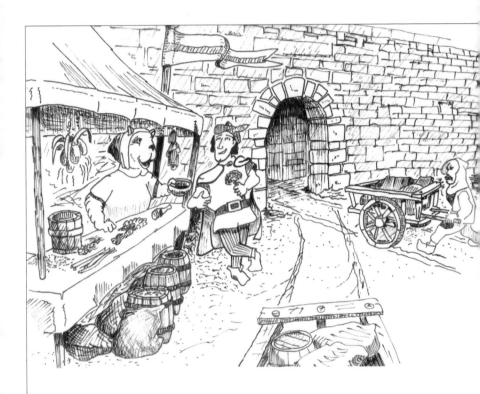

Horace captivated Heather with his eyes,
his looks, and his charm.

"And Heather," Wanda said, "our herb lady and Wellness Wombat, she saw this happening?"

"Yes," Warren said, clearly enjoying his storytelling role. "Heather saw the sales of herbs at her market stall drop and watched as medicine fought to intentionally gain public trust and position itself as the only alternative. Medicine had to replace the beliefs people had in folklore, alternative remedies, or prevention with the doctrine graduate students repeated and the science medical schools promoted: one that said people could no longer manage their health; medicine had to. Heather saw the awe people held for everything the emerging new medicine was doing. She saw people lose interest in the old ways, too, ways they had relied on to manage their health for years.

"But, our herb lady didn't want her mind conditioned like that now did she? She didn't want her body, or her turf, invaded either, or experimented on in the name of this new science. Heather wanted the right to heal herself with nature's herbs and plants, and not be told by practitioners prescribing alchemists' unnatural concoctions that their way was best. Heather was a Wellness Wombat. She was willing to care for her own health and eager to pass on the benefits of her proven natural alternatives. She was critical of the new medicine and its intentions to replace those alternatives.

"Heather had her critics, though," Warren continued. "Many of them were doctors-in-training at the medical school on the other side of the huge stone wall where she had her market stall. One of them stopped by her stall on his way to eat lunch one day and got her attention."

"What happened?" Rick said.

"Chemistry," Warren said with a grin. "His name was Horace. He captivated Heather with his eyes, his looks, and his charm and she fell in love. So, now there was conflict and a subtle tussle for power. Heather was a Wellness Wombat promoting healing potions in love with a medical student taught to use medicine's lotions and treat people in ways she didn't believe in."

"Interesting," Ed said, holding his glasses up to the light to clean them. "What happened?"

"She taught him about alternatives, of course! On romantic walks through the English countryside and on visits to the monastery herb gardens, Heather revealed the powers of the herbs and wildflowers she sold and told Horace how her potions worked. She took him away from the haze of the medical maze and let nature's ways amaze." Warren turned to Wanda. "You're the resident herb lady. Give us some examples of what Heather might have shown him."

"Be happy to. I've studied this stuff for years," Wanda quickly replied. "She would have shown him herbs like watercress and coriander for culinary use, or wild basil, nettle, or feverfew for medical use, such as a tea to loosen a chest cold. I still recommend it at my tea bar in the Spa to members with a chest cold. Our herb lady would have sold herbs for everyday use, too. People traveled by horseback then and like us in our cars, had accidents: broken collarbones, fractures and, of course, saddle sores. She would have sold them wild comfrey for setting bones; the root was pounded into a mash and spread around wooden splints. Or horseradish mixed with grease as a liniment to relieve pain. I'll bet she sold a lot of eryngo root too, the aromatic gum people chewed to guard against infection from plague."

"What about travelers in London who were getting upset stomachs from tavern food?" Warren asked. "What would she have sold for that?"

Wanda rattled off the answer. "Dandelions made into a tea were always good. Bayberry, devils claw, or goldenseal root, or herbs like catnip or skullcap all helped digestion. Oh, and slippery elm bark, for stomach acid. And while she strolled through the countryside with her boyfriend, she would have collected stuff local traders and merchants bought from her to make what they sold, like germander for brewing ale, or blackberry, bilberry, soapwort, tanner's root, and greenweed for dye."

"Wow," Rick said. "A far cry from the antacids and other synthetic drugs we rely on today. So she cured people with all that stuff?"

"More people than her doctor-to-be fiancée did," Warren replied. "The medical school taught Horace to go to the apothecary or, druggist. But he came around. He respected Heather's ways and avoided the ways of the maze so they could both take care of people's health in their own way. Horace still became a doctor, but practiced in the country, where he could combine Heather's remedies with his own knowledge."

Ed laughed. "Oh," he said. "So, they're an early example of integrated medicine."

"Horace is an early example of you, Ed," Wanda said enthusiastically "A frustrated medical practitioner critical of the doctrines he'd been taught and the ways of the medical maze. I bet Heather was happy she married a doctor, though, eh Warren? I bet he made more money providing the new medicine people wanted than she did selling herbs."

"Horace did make more money, but with Heather working beside him patients had a choice; the kind of choice more people want today. But, because of the doctrine I shared with you that medicine spread back then, Heather's practices were being questioned and Horace's embraced; even though Horace's methods still hadn't gained the trust Heather's had. Here's why. Medicine was battling a doctrine that was set in the fifteenth century and it went like this: Public Health Boards, in spite of their policy of encouraging the opening of medical schools, were created to keep the public *away* from doctors."

"Because of all the quacks toting their remedies during the plague," Ed suggested.

"That's right," Warren replied. "But you see the dilemma. Medicine, and its schools, wants to inoculate people with the doctrine that only they with their new medicine and science can manage the public health. Public Health Boards want to inject their doctrine that they are in charge of the health of the public."

"So, what happened?" Rick asked.

"Medical schools were forced to support the Public Health Boards' agenda and teach the public about hygiene and how to keep its water supply and streets clean. It didn't want the doctors the schools were dispensing to practice any quackery. Public Health Boards were set up to police the conditions in which people lived and to prevent those conditions from creating any more plagues. They were set up to police how quacks in both fields of medicine practiced, too.

"Here's where it gets interesting. In order to build its own institution, the medical maze we know today, and have its doctrines embraced, medicine had to patiently take shelter under the public health movement roof and abide by the rules it set. It had to convince the Public Health Boards, and a wary public, that it could be trusted with and given responsibility for the public's health one day. Medicine needed an endorsement from public health if it were to become powerful enough to break away to form its own association and manage the public's health. I'll explain how medicine broke away in Stage Eight, when I talk about modern public health practices.

"For now, let's just say that medicine succeeded. It slowly erased people's memories of the old ways and their reliance on Public Health Boards to police medicine's practices. And it injected the public with the doctrine that eventually spread through society as the social disease that we still suffer from today, one that has impacted more lives than any plague: the giving up of responsibility for one's health."

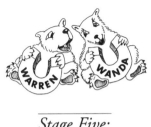

Stage Five:

The Bloodletter, the Body Snatcher and the Knife Grinder

"YOUR FOOD IS HERE!" GAIA ANNOUNCED CHEERFULLY AS SHE placed the lunch orders in front of everyone.

"Thank you," Warren said looking at his Body Snatcher sandwich. "Who's ready for another juice?"

"I've got room," Rick said patting his belly fondly and then pulling his plate closer.

"I do too," Wanda said.

"And me too!" Ed cried, inhaling the steam rising from his Witches Gruel soup.

"Be back as soon as I can," Gaia said heading off to get refills.

Rick, Wanda, and Ed eagerly started eating, but Warren continued to hold court.

"Okay," he said, leaning confidently forward with a warm smile. "The story I'm about to tell you is a little gruesome. It's set in the eighteenth century and it's about the bloodletter, the body snatcher, and the knife grinder. It's also about the illegal sale of human organs and other body parts which, to confirm my claim about medicine repeating its unhealthy patterns, is something that still takes place today.

"Anyway, this is an important stage in the construction of the medical maze. It's when the incision decision was made and because of it, the maze grew faster than a tumor. Doctors weren't just fighting for turf anymore; they were fighting for bodies. Cadavers; dead bodies! From the seventeen hundreds on, in London and Edinburgh especially, they were in high demand."

"Bodies were still being snatched up in the nineteenth century here," Ed said.

"Sometimes before they even hit the cemetery," Warren responded. "Anyway, while we're sinking our knives into our food, let's talk about physicians and anatomy students sinking their knives into people. It began in the thirteenth century when bloodletting was used to help restore health. Bloodletters cut veins open to bleed patients of toxins and reduce fevers, but many doctors let too much blood, killing the patient instead, and giving the medical profession a bad rap. Medicine and the public believed bloodletting worked. It worked for some and killed others, somewhat like radiation and chemotherapy do today. What can I say? Quackery was everywhere. It still is. And the incision decision set the stage for it."

Rick looked puzzled. "How?" he asked.

"Well, let's take anatomy, the art of dissecting the body to study it, as an example, and dissect medicine's beliefs about it. For centuries medicine based its practices on what a fellow named Galen, around 200 AD, drew. Drawings they religiously referred to as the bible of anatomy that, it was later discovered, were based on the anatomy of the ape. Don't worry. Even Leonardo Da Vinci screwed up. His sketches were based on animals he'd dissected also. In other words, doctors sliced and diced and made incision decisions using knowledge based on animal anatomy, and then passed those practices on through the medical schools to their students."

"Until 1538, when Versalius, a Belgian physician, corrected everyone," Doctor Ed added.

"That's right. Now you know, Rick, why it's important to understand the history behind the maze you got caught in, and to walk the middle path of self-care, where you take responsibility for your health and don't put it into the hands of either field of medicine. You see why quacks promoting natural remedies back then viewed medical students, eager to practice what they'd discovered about anatomy and how the body worked, as quacks too."

"There's no question," Ed said, "that early medicine in its haste to master nature, or at least dissect it, made a lot of mistakes. It was at the forefront of a new science which was then and is now, an unproven science."

"Its business is still about convincing people that only medicine can heal them," Warren said, fixing his gaze on Rick again. "In my opinion it's the incision decision that helped medicine strengthen their claim that the body was too complex for people to manage anymore. It helped medicine convince people to quit moving their own magnet by healing their body with nature's remedies and look to medicine for answers instead.

"For example, the old practice of bedside manner, where the patient was carefully diagnosed by a doctor who listened as his patient explained how he felt, was replaced by what science declared instead of what the patient shared. The outcome of that decision was that doctors were too eager to categorize their patient's condition so that they could practice

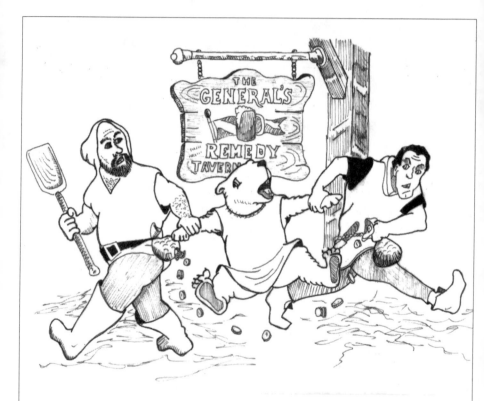

Things fell apart after Morgan, the body snatcher,
and Morris, the knife grinder, shared stories
with Mason at the local tavern.

science and its new surgical techniques. The patient ended up, secured by leather straps on an operating table, without anesthetic, in front of dozens of well-dressed medical students who watched each cut."

"And I'll bet your body snatcher sold the corpse back to those well-dressed students, if the patient died," Rick muttered.

"You can blame Herophilus of Chalcedon, the Greek physician, for the body snatcher mess," Warren explained. "You can thank him for the gaping wound he opened between nature-based healers and doctors, too. Herophilus was the founder of anatomy and, like Galen, he learned his art from dissecting animals not humans. But, he made the incision decision that put body snatchers in business.

"You see, Rick, the Greeks and the Romans originally viewed the body as sacred architecture and dissection of the human corpse was considered unethical. That all changed when the incision decision was made. Roman physicians didn't respect that view for long either once they had access to the chopped off parts of gladiators to help them learn about anatomy. Now you can see why a knife grinder was so popular. He had to keep surgeons on the cutting edge."

"So, tell us the story," Rick said impatiently.

Warren willingly returned to his story. "It begins with Mason, an eighteenth century bloodletter who killed more patients than he healed. To make money, so he could eat, Mason sold the bodies to his friend Morgan the body snatcher. Morgan sold them to medical schools, anatomy students, and eager surgeons. Surgeons needed sharp tools, to make their incision decisions, and stay ahead in the race for new medical discoveries about how the body worked. That's where Morris, the knife grinder, comes in. His body snatcher friend referred him to everybody."

"Isn't Mason the Wellness Wombat?"

"Yes, Wanda, he is. Mason's intentions were always to heal not hack, but he got caught up in the popular practices of his time. Bloodletting was one of them. Not one he was very good at, because he kept losing patients whom he sold to Morgan, his body snatcher friend, to save him the job of going to graveyards at night to dig them up. But, things fell apart after Morgan, the body snatcher and Morris, the knife grinder, began to share stories with Mason at the local tavern. Stories about the grizzly experiments taking place on the bodies of the patients he had sold them."

Ed smiled. "Many were cut on, but few survived."

"And it was all that cutting on that gave our Wellness Wombat bloodletter cause for concern. Mason felt bad, you see, about the people whose bodies he had sold, because he knew them before he unintentionally killed them with his bloodletting exercise. Mason decided he was in the wrong career, so he returned to his roots just as our wombats in Sydney did. He was disappointed with where medicine was going and its focus on offering convenience and short cuts. Mason wanted to return to nature's ways, not fuel the incision decision and the liberties medical science was taking with the bodies of his clients.

"Mason's decision affected Morgan, the body snatcher who had to go back to digging in graveyards at night because his supply had suddenly dried up. And Morris, the knife grinder, was affected also. His business was cut in half. The good news is that by turning back to natural medicine, our bloodletter Wellness Wombat helped more people. He refused to cut on anyone and rediscovered the powers of herbal remedies instead. Mason taught people how to take responsibility for their own health. Oh, he moved out of town too, and became a farmer to get away from the unhealthy air of authority doctors, and even bloodletters, were adopting then."

"Did the knife grinder stay in business?" Rick asked.

"He did. Body snatchers and knife grinders stayed in business right up to the nineteenth century when anatomy became a hot topic again.

"But I want to talk for a minute about the American Civil War, where knife-wielding Army surgeons took the incision decision to another level and kept knife grinders very busy. The art of bedside manner had no place in war. Pain of the wounded often had to be ignored. Surgeons on the battlefield relied on adrenaline to keep them going and on their skill with the knife to keep the wounded going. Eager to limit the pain that the soldiers suffered, surgeons dissected and amputated as fast as they could, unaware of the origins of the incision decision or any traditions that demanded respect for the body."

"A respect Hippocrates, the Greek physician, tried to retain when his band of self-proclaimed healers created the Hippocratic Oath around 400BC," Ed said.

"An oath that wasn't used in medical school until 1508 in Germany and one that few doctors use today," Warren countered. "The White Coat Ceremony is becoming more popular now. New medical students don the coat to signify entry into the elite ranks of their chosen profession, once again widening the gap and level of trust between doctor and patient. But, back to the battlefield: during the American Civil War most Army surgeons had entered medicine to help the sick get well, but many of them also saw the opportunity to make money and establish a reputation. So, they fought another battle at the same time, the establishing of their territory or, turf, the battle I shared with you earlier. Army surgeons carved out reputations for themselves by who could saw off the most limbs."

"With those freshly sharpened knives," Ed said, peering down over the top of his glasses.

"Speed counted?" Rick said, amazed. "Did skill?"

"With little access on the battlefield to anesthetics, the most compassionate surgery was the fastest. Fewer patients in pain meant a better reputation." Warren sunk his knife into his Body Snatcher sandwich for dramatic effect. "Sadly, most of the wounded died from post-op infection. But that didn't matter; status was measured on operating table results back then, not on the survival rate." He pulled the knife back out of his sandwich and looked up at Rick. "And, in today's maze, surgeons under stress from unrealistic workloads have to be swift with the knife too; too swift in fact, as they even cut on the wrong limb sometimes."

Gaia quietly placed the juice refills everyone had ordered on the table and left.

"So, Rick, I've called this stage the incision decision; a decision that began as a small cut, but over the centuries has become a torn and untended sore. It's a decision that still infects our present generation and will fester among future generations, too, if ignored."

"A great analogy, Warren, but it isn't doing much for my lunch," Rick remarked, making everyone laugh.

"Well, let me put it this way: other Wellness Wombats like Mason the bloodletter tried to protest the influence of the incision decision. They objected to the blatant race by medical practitioners to secure a reputation and a place in the medical maze. They tried to alert people to what was happening and encouraged them to ask: "Is this moving my magnet or is it helping me to move my own?" But, once again, Mason and the alternative medicine he was trying to promote, were suppressed by the advance of new traditions and the tactics that medicine employed to build its maze."

"Look at the bright side," Rick said, "if the incision decision hadn't been made, and the study of anatomy pursued, you wouldn't have a medical maze to dissect, would you?"

Everyone followed Warren's lead as he raised his glass. "Let's all drink to that, and give medicine the credit it deserves," he said, putting his glass back down. "Before the incision decision was made to help practitioners learn more about the body, they were just guessing how it worked. They know a lot more today and, with laparoscopic or endoscopic minimally invasive surgery, the incision is often less than two centimeters long. We've come full circle; the incision decisions doctors make now actually respect the body."

Wanda tossed her hair back. "Yes, but when you chart medicine's past, its unhealthy history, a ravenous desire to master nature and the living forms it sustains jumps out."

"I agree," Ed said. "Accepting stolen corpses from graveyards wasn't beyond medicine in the nineteenth century. Spiriting away their organs in the twenty-first century isn't either. Medicine still has an ego. I can certainly testify to that. It still sees the human body as experimental material, to be surgically refashioned, genetically manipulated, age-retarded, even cloned; and above all, to be mastered."

"To be drawn like a magnet, you mean, into the medical maze," Wanda remarked.

"Medicine can't pay body snatchers like Morgan anymore," Ed replied, "but anyone not moving his or her own magnet is subject to being pulled into the maze like a magnet. Medicine still wields its power and asserts its influence."

"I think Voltaire, one of my favorite eighteenth century French writers, summed it up best. He said, 'A doctor's job is to amuse the patient while nature cures the disease.' I keep saying it; people need to quit relying so much on medicine and start taking responsibility for their own health."

Rick winced slightly as he reached for his salad. "That's easy to say but hard to do."

"Well, enough of incision decisions," Warren declared. "Let's go to Stage Six in the construction of the medical maze, where doctors cut off what they needed most."

"Cut off what?" Rick asked, holding a forkful of salad.

Warren smiled. "Not what; whom?"

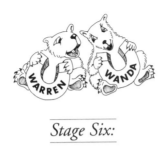

Stage Six:

The Nurse at the Camp with a Swinging Lamp

"THEY CUT WOMEN OFF," WARREN CONTINUED, CLEARING HIS throat slightly. "My story about Gwen and Godfrey, the medieval witch and woodcutter in Stage One, told how women who dared to claim they could treat the sick were treated by men eager to stake that claim themselves. It was the start of a long period of mistreatment of women in medicine. In the nineteenth century, where Stage Six takes place, doctors still upheld the arrogant attitude that their male ancestors had injected into medicine at its birth. Doctors cut women down verbally if they were already working in medicine as nurses, ignored the contributions they were making, and blocked their way if they dared to step on the path that led to a medical career. Even the Hippocratic Oath I just mentioned encourages the teaching of men, not women. So this story, Rick, is about the mistreatment of women in medicine, a tradition that men in medicine, even today, still uphold and enforce."

"Women got burned," Wanda declared angrily.

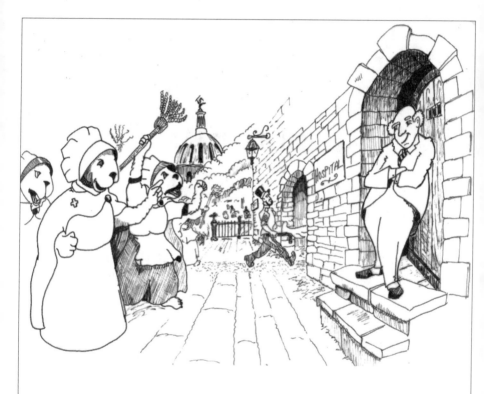

Florence Nightingale rallied the nurses to
fight for the right to practice medicine.

"They did," Warren agreed. "But let me introduce you to a lady who didn't. In fact she did the burning. She's my Wellness Wombat in Stage Six because she literally brought a breath of fresh air back into the world of medicine by bringing back nature and its elements. She had a huge impact on the construction of the medical maze and on public health policies."

"Thanks for the fresh air clue," Doctor Ed said. "You're talking about Florence Nightingale, the lady with the lamp, I presume?"

"The swinging lamp, Ed," Warren stressed. "Florence is the nurse at the camp with a swinging lamp. That's my title for this story. She swung her lamp in Crimean War Army Camps and burned boatloads of oil doing it. She should have slogged the doctors across their heads with her lamp for the way they were running army hospitals back then! Instead, tired of seeing so many wounded Crimean War soldiers die from infection, Florence Nightingale campaigned for better sanitation."

"Did you say infection?"

Warren laughed. "Yes, Rick. Our Wellness Wombat knew that the same sanitary practices the Romans had practiced saved parts of Europe from the Plague. She knew those same practices would save soldiers in her camps as well. And they did. In 1854, she returned to her native England as a hero. She had stormed the walls of the medical maze, battled the men defending the turf they had built it on, and fought against the quack ideas medicine had about treating the wounded and managing the sick."

"Quack ideas like keeping the sick cooped up in dark rooms with closed windows," Wanda said. "Only one of the lessons she took back to England, where everyone was already talking about the way she had marched right into wounded soldiers' rooms, shocking the Army doctors, and flung windows open to let in fresh air and light. She moved sick soldiers and their beds into tents outside to teach her proud know-it-all doctors how much healthier fresh air and open windows were than dark, stuffy, germ filled rooms. You can imagine how unsettled men in medicine were by her antics."

Rick shifted his weight again, trying to get comfortable. "I bet it just made them sick."

"She became a clot in medicine's bloody pool of nineteenth century progress," Warren replied. "I think her timing was perfect, though. She stirred surgeons up and made them earn their reputations by working harder to gain public trust. She helped nurses and surgeons' assistants gain some respect, too. Florence Nightingale put common sense back into the world of medicine at a time when it was building its maze on scientific quackery."

Doctor Ed's infectious smile cast its glow again. "She was much more than a nurse. She was a tireless campaigner who saved lives."

"In the midst of the Crimean War she fought her own war," Warren replied. "She rallied the other nurses into determined squads of women who scrubbed away infectious outdated thinking practices along with infection spreading bacteria. Her work at the Army hospitals made civilian hospitals cleaner and safer. She put compassion and heart back into medicine by reviving the ancient Greek practice of bedside manner proud nineteenth century doctors had discounted and replaced with science. She was a true Wellness Wombat. She practiced healthy disciplines and then, by word of mouth, spread the benefits of those disciplines to others.

"After the war, she returned to England and became an advocate for rural hygiene and sanitary reform. She taught country folks about sanitation, basic things like cleaning up cesspits and privies so they wouldn't infect the water supply and spread cholera. She knew that if you respected nature it would teach and heal you, so that medicine couldn't reach you and hack you."

"That's pretty dramatic," Rick said. "So, this stage is about women in general, or is it just about your lady with the lamp?"

Wanda shared her opinion. "This stage is about how medicine treated women while constructing their maze, Rick. It's about how women fought to regain the respect and position their ancestors once held. Their ancestors had to worry about not getting burned. The women Florence Nightingale was stirring up shared a burning desire."

"And now it was the medical practitioners' turn to worry about getting burned," Warren said, adding drama to his story. "Like soldiers gazing in disbelief at their own hemorrhaging wounds, doctors were in shock. The walls of their precious medical maze were under attack, threatened by the growing influence of women in medicine who were determined to loosen the tourniquet of authority that still held them captive."

"But women back then were expected to know their place, weren't they?" Rick asked.

"Not only know their place, but also keep quiet in it," Wanda declared bluntly. "Something women no longer have to do today and something Florence Nightingale didn't do then."

"Nor did the nurses she inspired," Warren added. "During the eighteen hundreds any female patient or nurse who questioned the authority of a male surgeon, no matter how insane his incision decision, was seen as a threat."

"And, in turn were threatened," Wanda said.

"There's more," Warren explained, "the incision decision opened the door to experimentation and not just for surgery, either. Around 1820, women, usually poor women who died from shock or infection later, were more often the subjects of those experiments. Women were poorly treated, not just as nurses, but as patients too.

"Women were welcome on the operating table, but were blatantly barred from admittance into medical schools until the 1840s, even in this country. That's why Florence Nightingale led the way and threw herself into nursing. It was the only way she could enter medicine."

"If only the men in medicine had treated the women eager to serve in medicine differently, patients might have received better treatment," Doctor Ed lamented.

"But even in big city hospitals they didn't necessarily get better treatment, Ed," Warren responded. "While hospitals were struggling to find ways to treat common ailments, savvy women from rural villages confidently applied inherited remedies that worked; old folklore traditions like boiling bark from back yard trees to cure stomach ailments was only one of them. The kind of alternatives hospitals couldn't use then, and still refuse to use today. The integrated medicine that we want today where practitioners in the medical maze embrace alternative remedies still has a long way to go.

"Anyway, back to Florence Nightingale," Warren said, using his deep voice again. "What I admire most about her is how she rallied women in medicine into action, women who were ready to be more than just pandering nurses who were persecuted for expressing their opinions. By promoting the same compassionate and common sense alternatives that had stopped plagues in the past, Nightingale made it possible for pioneers like Mary Walker, the first female doctor in America, and others like her to play the role in medicine that they do today.

"Florence Nightingale was a great Wellness Wombat," Warren concluded. "She believed a hospital should be a healthy place, free of infection, discrimination, and intimidation. She opened the door and made it possible for other women to follow. In fact, in 1860, she responded to the continuing mistreatment of women by men in medicine by opening a School of Nursing."

"For the women who couldn't penetrate the medical maze or bear its patronizing attitude," Wanda moaned.

Warren chuckled. "There were a few that did penetrate the maze, even before Florence Nightingale came along. One of them dressed as a man."

"That quacks me up!" Rick's belly shook as he laughed.

"Seriously! Let me tell you the story," Warren said. "It was in 1778. Her name was Deborah Samson, from Massachusetts. She spent three years in the American Revolution Army disguised as a man. She joined the British Army too, and became an officer and an admired surgeon. No one knew she was a woman until her autopsy."

"Women were tough," Ed said. "The harder medical men, army or not, tried to repel them from the walls of their medical maze the more they fought to get in."

"Even if they had to disguise themselves as men to do it," Rick said with a snigger.

"We have women doctors today," Warren continued, "but nurse practitioners are still held back by their male counterparts and have to fight for their rights. Most nurse practitioners are restricted to administering secondary care, not primary care, and are as frustrated by the incompetence of the doctors they serve as Florence Nightingale was."

"So, men continue to dominate medicine," Rick proposed.

"They always have," Warren claimed. "Despite my respect for Florence Nightingale, women were never the only gender with great bedside manner."

"Men as healers; that sounds interesting," Rick mused.

"The first hospitals were monasteries, Rick run, as you know, by men. And most of the monasteries relied on their herb gardens for remedies. In the sixteenth century, Henry VIII destroyed almost every monastery in England during his quest to establish his own church. The nunnery, or convent, then took over the role of caring for the sick. You are familiar with female midwives and male surgeons, but you probably don't know that by the 1750s there were more male midwives than female midwives delivering babies in people's homes. For years to come, the tradition that 'medicine is for men' had been inherited and dominated how the medical maze was structured.

"But, men defended their position, their medical maze. They defended it by building more walls in the form of Gentlemen's Clubs, Surgeons Clubs, Guilds, and Medical Associations, all places where women were not admitted."

"Discrimination works both ways," Wanda declared. "Women fought back, didn't they? They formed institutions where men were not admitted, like Florence Nightingale's School of Nursing."

Ed nodded in agreement. "And the Institute of Nurses, also formed by women unhappy with the way medicine treated them."

"Good memory, Ed, but let's get on to Stage Seven," Warren said firmly, determined to keep his story telling on track. "Stage Seven is about the formation of those Guilds and Associations men in medicine used to defend their position. And because of the role these Guilds played in the construction of the medical maze I'm going to jump back to the thirteenth century. My next story is a bloody one. And my next little Wellness Wombat is a barber-surgeon."

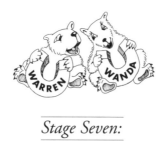

Stage Seven:

Red as Blood: White as Linen

"THIS STORY," WARREN BEGAN, "IS ABOUT HARVEY, A BARBER-surgeon apprentice who was as sharp as the knives he watched other barbers use, but less keen' to use them.

"It's set in thirteenth century London and, as part of his apprenticeship, our Wellness Wombat swept the bloodstained wooden shavings off the floor of his father's barbershop and hung the blood stained white linen bandages used as tourniquets to stop the bleeding outside the shop to dry. The red as blood and white as linen pole we associate with barber shops today wasn't used until later, but that's where the colors on the pole come from. The pole itself symbolizes the piece of wood customers squeezed in their hand so the barber could find a vein to cut into and bleed. It was also used to bite down on if a leg or an arm had to be sawed off. The blue on the pole symbolizes veins."

"So, what happens to our Wellness Wombat?" Rick wanted to know.

Warren leaned back in his chair and put both hands behind his head. "I already mentioned how insensitive to

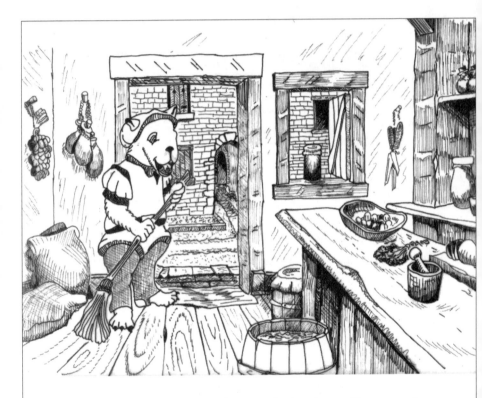

Harvey discovered that early barbers dispensed
herbal remedies to their patients before
they used sharp knives to draw blood.

their patient's pain doctors were trained to be. Well, Harvey's dad, William, was determined to make a man out of his son. Insensitive to Harvey's desires, William gave his son a knife, picked up a patient's arm and said, 'Bleed it.' Harvey was later forced to saw off limbs, too, but after seeing so many people come to such a bad end, he knew there had to be a better way than bleeding people to death or cutting off limbs."

"So, was he sharp enough to find that way and escape the medical maze?" Rick asked.

"Yes," Warren replied. "After studying the history of his craft, he discovered that early barbers dispensed herbal remedies to their patients before they used their sharp blades to let blood. Our Wellness Wombat was a barber before the barber-surgeons split up their guild and wanted nothing to do with surgery. So, he opened his own dispensary in a London suburb. He lined its shelves with bottles of herbal extracts, tinctures, and oils, and sold herbal remedies the way barbers used to do. He educated his customers about the benefits of a healthy lifestyle to keep them out of barbershops and away from surgeons and physicians."

Rick shifted restlessly in his chair. "So, barber-surgeons didn't just cut hair?"

"No. They let blood, pulled teeth, and severed limbs, too. You see, Rick, the early history of barbering reveals that barbers had as much respect in the tribe as the medicine men and the priests. So, it makes sense that after the church relieved monks of bloodletting and healing duties, barbers would be the logical choice.

"Let me give you all a quick history. Wanda hasn't even heard this one yet," Warren said as Wanda gave him a puzzled frown.

"In the Stone Age men used clam shells and flint to pluck hair and to shave. They got smarter and later used copper, bronze, and then iron razors sharpened with water and a whetstone, or a leather strop. The Egyptian barbers used razors that looked like small hatchets. The cut-throat steel straight razor was then followed by safety razors.

"Beard trimming was an art. Alexander the Great ordered his soldiers to have their beards trimmed because their enemies could grab them in hand-to-hand combat. The Latin word 'barba,' means beard. In the Dark Ages, the term barbarian described tribes who didn't shave. In Greece, while men's faces were being scarred by amateur barbers trimming their beards, women were singeing hair off their legs with a lamp."

"Ouch!" Wanda cried. "That must have hurt."

"Ouch, indeed," Warren said with a grin. "And, in eleventh century France, one Archbishop banned beards. The first barber organization that we know of was established in London in 1308, then later in the century, the first barber school was founded in Paris to teach the practice of surgery. Which brings me back to your question, Rick. Barber-surgeons didn't just cut hair; they made incision decisions, too. They were better known for cutting open veins on their patrons' arms and bleeding them into the blood collection bowls. The patients fainted of course, but barbers still competed for business with the best dentists and surgeons of the time."

"They would open a vein in the leg or neck as well as an arm," Doctor Ed quietly added. "They knew enough not to cut across and sever the vein, so they used a small knife called a lancet to cut along its length."

Rick shifted his weight into a more comfortable position before finishing the rest of his burger. "This is the second time you've talked about bloodletting, Warren. Why was it so popular?"

"Back then people believed disease was carried in the blood and had to be bled out. Today people believe it has to removed, but not by bloodletting. In medieval times, country folk were bled when they went to the market, to free them of evil diseases. It was a preventative practice. Later on, the wealthy practiced it, too."

Ed smiled again. "Barbers had the sharpest instruments in town so people went to them to be bled, Rick."

Warren nodded in agreement. "Most barbers were located near monasteries, Rick, where sick people went before there were hospitals. But monks were no longer allowed to let blood, pull teeth, or cut off limbs. Papal edicts in 1215 forbid them from coming into contact with contaminating body fluids. So, with some training, and even less knowledge, and no bedside manner, these practices were downgraded from surgery to craft status and given to barbers."

"Bloodletting, or phlebotomy," Doctor Ed explained, "began with the Greeks. It's been popular for over two thousand years, right up to the nineteenth century. The early doctors thought they could restore the balance of the blood and other body fluids, like bile and phlegm, by bloodletting."

Rick gave Warren a questioning look. "So barbers suddenly became surgeons?"

"Well, almost. They became barber-surgeons. Their newly acquired skills made them money, so they formed a Guild in 1450 to protect the right to practice. The same Barber-Surgeons Guild that Henry VIII sanctioned in 1540. Members were granted four hanged criminals every year to dissect and perform anatomy on, too. That's how barbers suddenly became both barbers and surgeons.

"The guild imposed standards and created apprenticeships for future barber-surgeons who eventually earned respect for their skills and the instruments they used to cut hair, lance boils, extract teeth, let blood, and even amputate arms and legs. But because barber-surgeons worked with their hands, not their brains, and there was no science behind their practice, they were looked down on by physicians as simple craftsmen who were just working a trade."

"But, in spite of opposition, the Barber-Surgeon Guild, supported by the ruling monarchs, held more power then than today's labor unions do. I think it was 1745, when it changed its name to The Company of Surgeons. Am I right?" Ed asked.

"You are. That was the year that marked the split when barbers became barbers and surgeons became surgeons. Barbers could no longer keep up with the advances being made in medicine, surgery, and dentistry. From that time on, barbers only cut hair and surgeons only performed surgery. Of course, most people today trust their barber. Few people in Harvey's time trusted medicine, despite the fact that doctors were gradually becoming more skilled. Natural healing and its alternatives were still fresh in their minds. It's not as fresh in the twenty-first century. Now medicine has a stronger hold."

"Didn't George Washington die because his physician bled him too much?" Wanda asked.

"Yes, in 1799," Warren replied. "He had a throat infection and died from it at the age of sixty-seven after being drained of nine pints of blood in one day."

"Nine pints; that's over half his blood!" Ed exclaimed. "And the practice of bloodletting still didn't get banned until eighty years later."

"My stars," Rick replied. "People were still bloodletting from the thirteenth to the nineteenth century? It took that long to change their minds?"

"So you can imagine how many years it's going to take the Wellness Wombats to get people like you to change theirs," Warren teased. "To change their beliefs about the relevance of the medical maze, I mean, and change their negative habits to positive ones. To be more alert to the ways of the maze and take responsibility for their health again."

"I know," Rick said, "to move their own magnets!"

"Okay, this stage in the construction of the medical maze is about medical men who both defended their position in the maze, and defended the walls of that maze from anyone practicing alternatives who could be scaling it. Their strategy was to build more walls in the form of Gentlemen's Clubs, Surgeons Clubs, Guilds, and Medical Associations, all places where women were not admitted. Now, the next phase is fairly predictable. As more Guilds and Associations were formed, primarily to hold their practitioners accountable, medicine became stronger and Public Health Boards became weaker."

"Pharmacists formed a guild as early as 1240 to monitor their members," Ed said, adjusting his glasses again. "The American Medical Association was formed to monitor its members and protect public health. It just went too far when it decided that the best way to protect the public was by taking every chance it could to expose alternative practitioners as quacks."

"The AMA? Hold on," Rick said, "aren't we jumping centuries here?"

"Sorry. Yes we are, countries, too. By the nineteenth century, changes in medicine were spurting across the States faster than blood from a severed artery," Warren said as he took another sip of juice. "Ed's right. The American Medical Association was established in 1847. In my opinion, it was set up so that medicine could do what every other guild or association had done before them: take control of the profession and position it. Not just to serve the interests of the public, but to serve their own. To do that, the American Medical Association needed to out flank and out rank public health first."

"Get out from under its roof, you mean?"

"That's right, Rick," Warren said enthusiastically, "the public health roof it had to take shelter under that I mentioned in Stage Four. Medicine did get out from under it and in time even became a respected and trusted body, a modern guild."

Doctor Ed wasn't so diplomatic. "It became a bully, you mean. A dictator, instead of a protector of public health."

"Don't look so surprised, Rick," Warren said. "The AMA's strategy and power upset its members, the public, and our government. It was convicted in federal court once in the nineteen thirties and twice in the nineteen eighties: for arrogantly repeating its unhealthy history of harassing and conspiring to suppress anyone practicing anything that offered the public an alternative to the medical maze it was building."

Rick still looked surprised. "They were convicted three times?"

"Yes. The most famous case was in 1987, when the AMA was convicted of trying to put the chiropractic profession out of business. About twenty years earlier it had formed a Committee on Quackery."

"But even after government officials got involved," Ed said, "the AMA didn't lose its power. It still dictates its terms to Public Health Boards today."

"So medicine won and the public lost?" Rick said, idly playing with the rest of his spinach salad. "That's scary."

"It is," Warren agreed.

"Especially when you have to work with it every day, like me," Ed said, putting his glasses back on.

"The public never had a chance," Warren said. "The Public Health Boards didn't either. They didn't have the funds medicine had, so they couldn't promote themselves on the same level that medicine did. It was during the Industrial Revolution that medicine learned how to sell itself, the same way other emerging new industries did by using Public Relations and marketing tools. You see, public health wasn't motivated by profit in the same way that medicine was, and still is, today."

"So, the medical maze got its way," Ed concluded. "It forced Public Health Boards, originally formed to help people avoid doctors, to promote it instead."

Warren reached for his juice again. "It was an absolute betrayal of the trust the public had finally put in medicine and of the trust they had put in Public Health Boards. It was an unsettling exchange of power, which quelled the growth of alternative practitioners and swelled the ranks of medical ones. The very reason the medical maze was built."

"And the witches burned," Wanda quietly added.

All Rick could say was, "Really? I never realized until now how much the American Medical Association felt so threatened by alternative medicine."

"It still feels threatened," Warren replied. "Why do you think it takes members who want to incorporate alternative medicine into their practice to task and reprimands them?"

"It will feel the threat again once the Wellness Wombats get mobilized and are seen as a force in the community," Wanda cried, "when enough parents and kids decide to act like Wellness Wombats and take their health back into their own hands."

Rick's laugh was a little nervous. "Well, if my experience is an example of what happens when you put yourself in medicine's hands, I'm not surprised people are frustrated and looking for alternatives. And have been for centuries, by the sound of it. So, you talked about medieval public health in Stage Four. Is modern public health next?"

Warren nodded. "I'm going to show you how nineteenth century medicine finally outranked and broke away from the Public Health Boards."

"Immobilized them, you mean, so they could better manipulate the public into swallowing what they were dispensing." Ed said.

"That's what Stage Eight is about," Warren said. "I call it The Water Worker, but it could just as well be called How the Public Health System Failed to Meet the People's Needs."

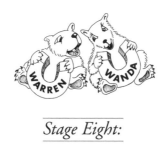

Stage Eight:

The Water Worker

"OUR WELLNESS WOMBAT IN THIS STORY IS SHERMAN," Warren said, enjoying the tales he was sharing. "Sherman's father was a prominent preacher and his mother a respected midwife. They raised him well; that's how he became a Wellness Wombat. Sherman is a health worker on the Public Health Board's payroll in nineteenth century London during the peak of the Industrial Revolution. Sherman's job is to preach the benefits of sanitation and clean water to the working class. I call him my water worker, and I guess that today he'd be the guy working for the Department of Public Health testing and maintaining water quality. Part of Sherman's job was to go to the unsanitary and overcrowded slums to educate poor factory workers about the importance of keeping clean. Sherman knew how important his job was but the Public Health Board he worked for didn't, not until after the damage was done, that is."

"What damage?" Rick asked brushing crumbs from his burger off his belly.

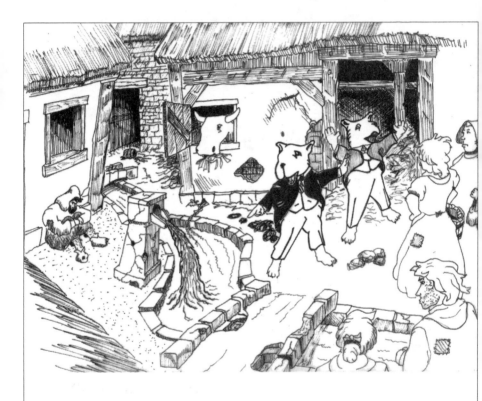

Sherman and his friend, John Snow, had to find
the source of the cholera outbreak and alert others.

"The damage to the population, the public health system, and the damage caused by the 1831 London cholera epidemic. The public health system failed to manage the epidemic, and the public lost trust in public health. There were riots in the streets," Warren said, gesturing enthusiastically with both hands. "Remember how in Stage Three, Europe's medieval public health system had forced sanitary practices on its crowded cities after the devastation of the plagues. Its modern public health system tried to impose healthier standards as well, but failed. Naturally, people took a closer look at what medicine was offering instead. Medicine then opened its doors wider, and drew people into its maze."

"Was there really a riot?" Wanda asked.

"There was indeed," Warren emphasized. "In fact, there were three major riots in less than twenty years. The job our Wellness Wombat water worker did suddenly became very important. He had to find the source of the cholera outbreak. And he did. In 1854 Sherman and his friend John Snow, a fellow wellness advocate, physician, and avid supporter of public health, traced the source of the cholera outbreak back to a water pump people were drinking from that was located next to some cowsheds and slaughterhouses. As you might guess, greedy merchants weren't inclined to provide sanitary conditions for their workers back then, or tell them how disease could be spread by waterborne parasites from the open sewage pits near their only water supply."

Warren raised his glass. "Cheers, Rick. Here's to our Wellness Wombat who drank beer back then because it was safer than water. The water was contaminated. Something that was ignored despite the many warnings Sherman and John Snow issued to those who kept drinking water from the contaminated pump.

"My guess is that the convenience of having water overrode the possible effects drinking it might have, just as the convenience of consuming the junk food and sugar-laden sodas Main Street restaurants keep dispensing today overrides the possibility that those foods can make people sick."

"So, you were saying, the public had lost their trust in public health?"

"Yes, Rick, and that trust was never fully restored. Public health advocates, like Sherman our water worker, tried to regain that trust by improving the appalling conditions that greedy Industrial Revolution merchants in England had created. But they had a challenge. Poor health was the result of poor habits and lack of knowledge. Those habits had to change and people had to take responsibility for changing them which was something few people were willing to do."

"Sounds like your theme again," Rick said, with a sly grin.

"It is, and with medicine waiting in the wings to relieve people of taking responsibility for their health, changing unhealthy habits just because the public health system couldn't support the outcome of those habits, became unnecessary. It was obvious that Public Health Boards couldn't manage its responsibilities; they were plagued, if you'll pardon the pun, by the diseases population growth in cities bred and spread.

"Medical science, eager to get out from under the roof of the Public Health Boards so it could manage public health, kept demonstrating how ready it was to step in. It claimed it could defeat many diseases, and to master the microbes and bacteria spreading them. So, naturally people began to rely on medicine more and more and trust public health less."

"And deliberately get led away from alternative remedies again," Wanda reminded them.

"To sum up the relevance of this stage in the construction

of the maze, I'll say this: public health lost control. Medicine took control. People lost faith in the former and gained faith in the latter."

"It's no wonder," Ed said with a chuckle. "Medicine deliberately spent more time securing its position, and strengthening the cast of its medical maze than it did in doing the work Public Health Boards had invited it to do which was teaching the public how to avoid getting sick."

"That's right," Warren agreed. "Medicine was in the power seat now and it ignored the controls public health departments wanted to impose upon it and set out instead to dazzle the public with its scientific discoveries. But it didn't just dazzle them; it blinded them to the benefits that their unscientific nature-based health plan had been giving them for centuries. And it blinded them to how determined medical science was to not only replacing that reliance on nature, but master nature along the way."

"Science deserves some credit," Ed declared. "It did give us antiseptics, penicillin, anesthesia, and X-rays. It detected the microbe that causes tuberculosis, and discovered the bacteria responsible for staph infections. It discovered the causes of typhoid, influenza, and cholera, too."

"Great discoveries," Warren said, "but they helped convince the public that they should put their trust in medicine, instead of practicing the disciplines that taking responsibility for one's own health requires. Discoveries that deliberately diverted public attention, and turned people's heads away from healthy practices towards what doctors practiced instead."

"Toward what medicine was selling," Wanda added.

"This was a turning point," Warren claimed. "People didn't understand what was going on and, in fact, Public Health Boards didn't either. Medical science intimidated everyone.

No one knew enough to enforce or control how medicine was being practiced, or how to keep medicine, public health, and alternative care under the same roof. You might say that medicine's influence on public health spread like a virus and the influence public health had, dropped like a fever."

"Sounds like somebody's magnet was being moved," Rick said, adjusting his belt to make it looser.

"Thanks for the endorsement," Wanda said brushing her hair back away from her face.

"You're welcome," Rick mumbled, still looking at the noticeable overlap above his belt. "So, Warren, what happened to Sherman, our Wellness Wombat?"

"Oh, he sailed to New York City, to work for the Public Health Board there. He'd learned enough about taming cholera in London. It was time now, to learn about Yellow Fever."

"New York suffered from Yellow Fever every year, didn't it, Warren?" Ed asked.

"That's right. President John Adams didn't sign the Bill that let States form their own Public Health Boards and give them the power to police and manage their own public health until 1798. That's when the worst case hit."

Warren glanced around the table. "America had its plagues, or fevers, as we prefer to refer to them, and they eventually led to the formation of Public Health Boards. But a lot of these boards went the same way that the health board in London did; they had to step aside and let medicine manage public health. As Sherman had learned, medicine had blinded people with its science and drawn them into its maze, a maze that he as a Wellness Wombat was determined not to enter."

"A maze that medicine was able to practice its science in and strengthen, now that it had outranked and broken away from the Public Health Boards," Doctor Ed confirmed.

"And it was that scientific knowledge that put a medicine now free of the quack label exactly where it wanted to be: back in charge of the public's health. The construction of the medical maze was almost complete," Warren concluded.

"At the beginning of this impatient history, medicine took control of public health by burning witches. Now it burned the public again by wrestling control away from the Public Health Boards. Will it ever end?" Wanda asked.

"Oh, it gets worse. Stage Nine is about medical schools, the same ones medieval Public Health Boards started back in Stage Three. These schools and guilds matured during the modern public health era. They grew up to become colleges of medicine and medical associations."

"Is Stage Nine the final stage of construction for the medical maze?" Rick questioned.

"Not quite. This phase is about a part of medicine's history that most people aren't aware of though," Warren replied. "How medical colleges and schools provided fast and easy certification to churn out doctors, doctors who were certified to do no more than practice the new science of medicine they had just learned on an increasingly trusting and receptive public, a public blind to how self-reliant they once were on nature to keep them healthy and how reliant on medicine they were now becoming."

"A behavior doctors in the medical maze still question," Ed said seriously.

"And a doctor is my next Wellness Wombat. He questioned the blueprint the medical maze was based on, too," Warren announced.

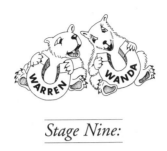

Stage Nine:

The Doctor's Rush for a Healthy Constitution

"THE DOCTOR WAS AN AMERICAN. HE STUDIED IN EDINBURGH and London before setting up a practice in late eighteenth century Philadelphia. He taught chemistry at one of the many medical colleges there, too. In Philadelphia, medical science was king. The town had a huge influence on the growth of medicine and was a magnet for medical students."

Warren looked at Rick to be sure he had his attention. "I've picked the doctor as my Wellness Wombat because he was one of America's greatest advocates of preventative medicine and proper diet. And he's a great example of everything we promote today. He questioned and tried to reduce the influence medicine was having. He believed medicine needed controls and that medical schools of the time, busy giving tools to fools, were doing more harm than good. His actions reveal the role medical schools had back then in our next phase of the maze."

"Is this the guy who opened the first free dispensary?"

"You guessed it, Ed," Warren replied.

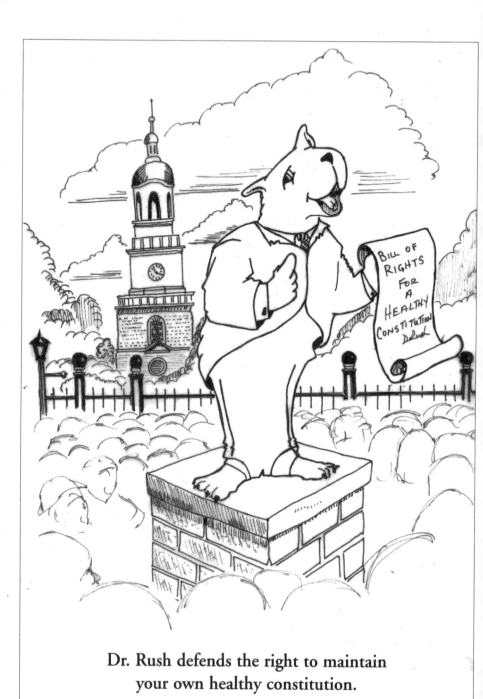

**Dr. Rush defends the right to maintain
your own healthy constitution.**

"So it's Benjamin Rush."

"Hey! He's the guy in stage one," Rick said. "What did he say again? That if medical freedom wasn't put into the Constitution…"

"Medicine would organize itself into an undercover dictatorship," Warren finished.

"So, this wombat was a bit of a fighter, in medicine but not sold on it. A little bit like you, Ed," Rick observed.

"Benjamin Rush was one of many throughout the history of medicine who questioned what medicine was doing," Warren explained. "Paracelsus, who taught at a sixteenth century university, was also a chemist. He actually burned books written by respected medical authorities because he claimed that they were full of quackery. He thought it was scandalous that doctors encouraged people to spend money on foreign substances and foreign procedures when the herbs in their back yards would have helped them just as much."

"How about Oliver Wendell Holmes Senior, the Boston physician who criticized his own profession?" Ed asked. "He said: 'Medicine would be better off, but the fish would be worse off, if every drug medicine dispensed was sunk to the bottom of the sea.' About 1860, I think it was."

Warren grinned. "You see, Rick, there have been critics inside the medical maze throughout every stage of its construction, questioning the trust the public places on their profession. And, as you said, Doctor Ed is ours."

"Thanks," Ed said, pretending not to notice the compliment. "But I haven't quite made the impact on medicine that Dr. Rush did. He helped cure the people of Philadelphia of Yellow Fever, you know."

"That's right, in 1793," Warren said, seizing the chance to delve into another segment of history. "He dismissed other doctors as quacks because they claimed that since the epidemic was airborne there was no cure. Dr. Rush used laxatives, cold baths, hot barley water, and other remedies to treat people. Remedies few paid heed to, though. There was another epidemic six years later. That one scared the public health authorities so much that even they fled to the countryside to escape it. But Dr. Rush stayed in the city and cured people, and then got criticized by other doctors for doing so. But, his beliefs about medicine becoming a dictatorship, if the right to freely choose how we manage our own health were not added to the Constitution, are still quoted today. The man was a true Wellness Wombat. By word of mouth, he established his reputation and, by word of mouth, he alerted the public to medicine's ways."

Warren paused. "I guess you could say he made people question the ethics of medicine and the rush it was in to license so many doctors at new medical schools popping up everywhere. Many of those schools were built to support science-based medicine's goal of replacing holistic medicine by quickly granting licenses. Doctors were determined to shed their old sawbones and quacks image, an image others probably even had of Dr. Rush because of his belief in bloodletting, but an image quickly erased by the work he did fighting Yellow Fever and the ways of the maze until he died in 1813."

"It wasn't until after he died, that the government finally stepped in to support his ideas about imposing controls on medicine and medical schools. Am I right?"

"Yes, Ed, you're right. The government had to step in. It had to slow the rapid growth of medical schools that began around 1765 that were approved to license doctors and was now getting out of control." Warren looked at Rick. "Back then most medical schools were privately owned by business savvy doctors who were less concerned about the quality of their graduates and more concerned about the number of apprentices they churned out. In the eighteenth century only about one in nine students could afford to go abroad to seek an approved degree. The rest had to get their medical training at one of the newly created medical schools here."

"Tell me more about Dr. Rush," Rick asked.

"Glad to. Dr. Rush had many allies; one of them was John Morgan, another American. Like Dr. Rush, John Morgan knew that standards for medical school apprentices were lax. He wanted standards set and exams passed for licensure. The government did step in to try and implement controls on the medical school business, but it wasn't until it sponsored the Flexner Report in 1910, that these controls were finally implemented. Controls that approved and certified medical schools run by universities and disapproved of medical schools run as businesses."

"True, the Flexner Report succeeded in limiting the number of doctors available," Ed said thoughtfully stroking his beard, "but it also increased their status and income. It produced less quantity and more quality at a time when demand for and trust of medicine was increasing."

"Did becoming a doctor mean you automatically made money?" Rick wondered.

"Absolutely not. And I have a great example," Warren quickly replied, "Sir Arthur Conan Doyle who wrote the Sherlock Holmes books; he was practicing medicine in London, but found it so competitive that he had to write books to pay his bills. I think he got lucky. His success as a writer meant that he could give up his medical practice. Many of our doctors are just as disillusioned with how medicine is managed today; they write or collect consulting fees to supplement income that managed care has cut in half."

"Or worse, they pay off the debt they exchanged for a medical degree by pushing the pills drug companies promote and become part of the great drug-vending machine we call medicine today," Ed said with a tinge of sarcasm.

Warren raised his index finger. "Say, that reminds me of Voltaire, the French writer I mentioned earlier, who said: 'Doctor's poured drugs of which they knew little to cure diseases of which they knew less into people about whom they knew nothing.' I love that quote."

"And my response to it," Ed said, clearing his throat, "is that we know more about curing disease today and more about how the person we are pouring drugs into functions. But we still don't know enough about how the drugs we are prescribing really work."

"People are just as likely to quit taking those drugs as they are to ask themselves, 'Who moved my magnet?'" Rick said as he shifted in his chair again. "You move people's drugs out of the medical maze and they'll be scurrying around that maze asking, 'Who moved my doctor's phone number? Who moved my emergency room? Who moved my medications and my drive-thru pharmacy?' long before they think to ask, 'who moved my magnet?'"

"What about you, then, Rick?" Warren asked. "After everything my Wellness Wombats have shown you, aren't you wondering who moved your magnet?"

"After listening to your engaging version of medicine's history, you bet I am." Rick fidgeted a little nervously with the napkin that was still tucked into his shirt. "Becoming a Wellness Wombat sounds like a fun way to get on the path to wellness and I know that healthy ways will keep me out of the maze. I just don't know if I have what it takes to practice them."

Ed gave him a friendly nudge. "We understand, but if you want to avoid getting caught in the medical trap again you'll have to change your old negative habits and make room for new positive ones."

"You said you wanted to live long enough to see your grandchildren. Why not try Warren's Wellness Wombat idea?" Wanda proposed. "Check out total health and see how feeling good feels for a change. I'll even give you a free pass to my Health Club and Spa to get you started."

Warren interrupted. "Hey, Rick. We understand your hesitation. Change is never easy. It's your choice whether or not you take responsibility for your health. You have to decide how consumed you want to be in the medical maze, so tell you what. Listen to Stage Ten and meet Sheila, my last Wellness Wombat. She's eager to wake you up to the consuming ways of the medical maze, and show you why you should manage your own health, and not expect medicine to do it for you anymore."

"A message we hope you'll take to your children one day," Wanda said.

Rick laughed nervously. "So they'll be like your kid? And spread the word about wellness? Being a Wellness Wombat probably isn't in the cards for my kids. I can't see them sharing the moral behind your Sydney rest stop tragedy with their school friends any time in their near future."

"If parents won't tell their kids how important it is to think differently about how their health is managed, then we have to hope children will take that responsibility for themselves," Wanda responded. "Joey's a bright child, and he's not shy. I bet he's got an audience right now, listening to another version of medicine's unhealthy history and the role the Wellness Wombats play in it."

Warren looked at Rick with a just-got-caught-with-my-fist-in-the-cookie-jar kind of grin. "Yeah. Just as Dad does every time he talks about the maze, sorry, the mess, we call healthcare. The mess Dr. Rush foresaw the public would get stuck with one day, where the public health model gets run into the ground by a more powerful profit-driven one."

Wanda sighed loudly. "But, his message got stashed away behind the walls of the maze like the medical records of a badly handled case, didn't it? Two hundred years later, we're still unhappy with the way medicine treats us."

"You know, I don't think the Burrows family will be the sole supporters of the Wellness Wombat idea for long," Ed said slowly. "This will spread. It has to. Some states are going bankrupt because they are spending more money on Medicaid than they are on educating their kids. The next generation will be a healthier one if we can start teaching kids to change their ways and stay out of the maze. Children have to take responsibility for their health, not expect social or insurance programs to tend to them when they get sick."

"Ed's right," Warren agreed. "If parents and kids in every community were to take our idea and see the fun that they could have in becoming healthy and sharing the benefits of good health by becoming Wellness Wombats, they could help break the repetitive patterns behind the history that built this maze."

Warren leaned forward and looked deep into Rick's eyes. "Your unhealthy habits moved you into the medical maze, Rick. If your kids inherit the same habits, they'll be moved, too. Not just moved, but consumed. Alternative medicine will be consumed as well.

And that brings me to Stage Ten: my final story. It's all about consumption and how medicine cemented the model we call healthcare into the consumer's mind. But, I'll let Sheila the wide-eyed wombat tell us all about that."

"Sheila?" Rick questioned. "Isn't that the name the Australians use for a woman?"

Warren laughed. "Yes, it is. Sheila goes to Australia at the end of the story to be with her relatives. It's my way of stressing how important it is to recognize the unhealthy cycles of medicine's repetitive history that I've just shared with you, so you won't get caught up in them. It brings my story full circle and back to where the Wellness Wombats began. Oh, we're in the early nineteenth century now, a few years after Dr. Rush died."

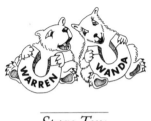

Stage Ten:

Sheila the Wide-eyed Wombat

WARREN SPUN HIS FINAL STORY. "SHEILA IS WIDE-EYED BECAUSE she saw her Mom's magnet was moved through the medical maze when she fell ill. Sheila and her mother worked at a textile mill near Boston. Sheila's eyes were opened after she saw how the medicine and the treatments that the quack doctors used on her mother to heal her actually killed her instead."

"Doctors the medical schools churned out in droves, the ones you talked about earlier," Ed remarked.

"Medical schools of the day taught their students to diagnose people like Sheila's mother by tasting their urine, treating them with foul-tasting concoctions that forced them to throw up, and then to bleed them to death; practices that were as accepted back then, as radiation and unproven medications are today. Sheila didn't trust the ways of the maze. Like any health-conscious, self-respecting citizen, she kept her eyes open. Her Mom's death opened them even wider, and spurred her on to become an active Wellness Wombat.

"You see, Sheila knew that if she had insisted that her Mom stay on the farm instead of moving to the city because there was work there, they would have used natural remedies to cure her when she got sick and not put their trust in the claims city quacks made. After Sheila's Mom died, she swore she'd never trust a doctor again. She became skeptical of everything, not just the new science of medicine that literally consumed her mother, but of anything new."

Warren focused his attention on Rick again. "I use the word consumed deliberately because Stage Ten is about consumption. There were two forms of consumption in the nineteenth century: the disease of consumption, also known as tuberculosis, which literally consumed the body; and consumerism, which consumed society. Sheila was really wide-eyed after she realized medicine had deliberately set out to consume others with their quackery and draw them, as they had drawn her mother, into its maze.

She saw how medicine changed the way people thought about how their health was managed and how inconvenient medicine made looking for alternatives sound."

"Is Sheila so wide-eyed because she's impressed, or scared?"

"Scared, Ed," Warren replied, "just as our friend Rick here is scared. Scared to change the habits that put him here today."

"I'm not scared," Rick said in quick defense. "I'm just not sure about all the alternative stuff *you're* consuming."

"One day this alternative stuff we eat and take to stay well will be mainstream, Rick," Wanda said. "And if you don't see that happening then you'll be wide-eyed, like Sheila, not because of the deceiving practices medicine employs but because of the huge number of people demanding alternatives to the medical maze."

"I might be one of those people," Rick mumbled. "So, tell me what happened to Sheila."

Warren smiled warmly and relaxed again. "Well, like the true Wellness Wombat she was, whenever she was asked, she shared the benefits of choosing a healthier path. Sheila grew up in the country so she was used to relying on her own or on her Mom's natural healing traditions and remedies. In the crowded city where people couldn't always afford to buy or find the time to pick the necessary ingredients they had relied on in the past for healing, Sheila found ways to make that happen. She had a fight on her hands though. Fewer and fewer people became interested in applying alternatives. Most became mesmerized by what medicine was selling.

"In a way, it was hard not to be. The Industrial Revolution was in full swing. People were getting consumed, not just by medicine, but by merchants, too. Merchants were now manufacturing and selling the same kind of soap, pottery, and textiles that people had made for themselves when they lived in the country. It was a great strategy. Merchant's lured people away from relying on making things for themselves and medicine lured them away from healing themselves.

"And our Wellness Wombat watched it all happen. She watched her Boston community give up the traditions of self-care and replace them with medicine's emerging model of healthcare. She watched as people were drawn, like magnets, from the country into the city by the promise of work, and from self-care to healthcare by the promise that it required no work.

"Before Sheila's Mom died, the textile mill where she worked provided only crowded cramped conditions, poor diet, soot-filled air, and contaminated water. These deplorable conditions fed people directly into the medical

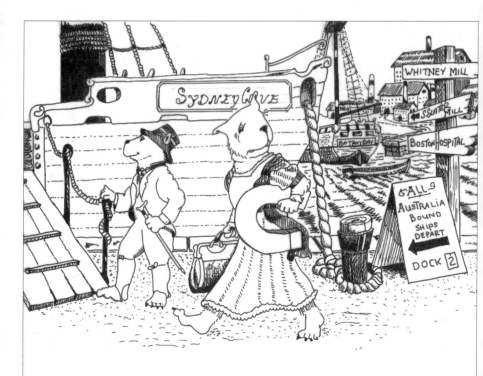

After seeing how consumed people were by the
medical maze, Sheila persuaded her husband
to move to Australia.

maze and into the hands of the newly certified doctors who were spilling out of the loosely governed medical schools I talked about earlier."

Wanda laughed suddenly. "You know, Sheila would be just as alarmed at the conditions modern day consumers tolerate today; the cramped cubicles, poor diets, polluted air, and contaminated water. Workers today aren't much better off than the workers Sheila and her Mom hung out with."

"That's something to think about. So, why were living conditions so bad back then?" Rick asked.

"I'm happy to answer that," Warren said. "Because this was the Industrial Revolution and greedy factory owners wouldn't spend their money on better housing for workers. This was the era of consumption: the consumption that made people cough up blood and the mass consumption that swayed people to cough up their money, too. It was a marketing age, and merchants had an easy market to sell to: the hordes of people crowding into the cities.

"That's the point of Stage Ten, to point out how medicine used these emerging marketing and sales tactics to cement the ways of the maze into people's minds. They sold people on using traditional medicine as an alternative to the country remedies they knew were now unavailable in the city. They sold them on unnecessary quack medical procedures too, just as they do today. That's how Sheila's Mom died. But, Sheila was determined not to die the same way, at the hands of so-called medicine. She may have been wide-eyed at the tactics medicine used to market themselves as the healthcare alternative to everyone moving into Boston territory, but she was still a Wellness Wombat and she took responsibility for her own health now. She didn't trust medicine with that, remember?"

"So, you said she moved to Australia?" Wanda asked.

"That's right, but not until after her Mom died. She went back to work at the mill first, where she opened the eyes of the mill owner in a very different way. He was wide-eyed at her beauty and he married her. They lived in a small country house, where there was plenty of fresh air and little chance of getting consumption or being consumed by the medical maze. She could pick the herbs she needed for remedies again and teach her husband about healthier ways than those of the maze.

"Years later, after seeing how industrialized America had become, how consumed the public was by the healthcare maze, and how well medicine's marketing machine worked, she persuaded her husband to move to Australia; to Sydney, in fact, where she taught others the lessons she had learned about taking responsibility for your own health and not getting consumed by convenient but unhealthy alternatives."

"If Sheila were still alive today she would be shocked at how consuming the medical model has become," Wanda said. "How securely it has cemented itself in the minds of consumers, who walk around with their eyes closed to how consumed they have become, and how many of their health rights and responsibilities have been taken away."

"More people are opening their eyes today," Ed said. "They see the cracks in the walls of the medical maze and want a healthier model. They're ready to become Wellness Wombats."

Rick laughed. "That is if you can divert their attention away long enough from the latest car, phone, or electronic gadget, to learn how to become one."

"If the Wellness Wombats catch on, and parents and children see them as a reminder that healthy ways keep you out of the maze, then the attention will be on education, won't it?" Wanda said, pushing her long black hair out of her face again. "Then the people you're talking about can use their electronic gadgets to get the information they need to be able to move their magnets. Or they could go to places like Quackers that cater to the wellness crowd, and visit their ER, their education room.

"Either one of those activities will consume their time in a healthy way." Wanda looked at Rick. "Anyway, I think we've said enough about consumption and the consuming influence of medicine. I want to hear your comments about Warren's ten stages."

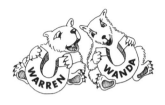

The Last Cut

WARREN FLOPPED BACK IN HIS CHAIR WITH HIS JUICE IN hand. "I think we all want to hear your comments. Besides, your walk with the Wellness Wombats through the history of medicine is over. At least with me it is. I hope it opened your eyes."

"Enough to know that I've got to make healthier choices than the ones that put me in the hospital," Rick said.

"And share what you've learned with others," Warren said, "so they'll see how important it is to practice healthy ways."

"Look, I know I've been skeptical about all this alternative stuff."

Warren smiled warmly. "Resistant, would be a better word."

"Okay, resistant," Rick agreed with a shrug of his shoulders. "Which is why you shared your bullet point history of medicine, I know. Look, I love the Wellness Wombats. I just don't see me becoming one right away. I'm not into all this health stuff the way you guys are. I probably will change my ways one day. I've got to if I want to stay out of the maze. But right now, I have to digest everything you've told me about how consumed I've been by medicine."

"See it for the prescription it is, Rick," Ed said. "One you can take—or not take."

"I know. Depending on how badly I want out. And I do want out, believe me. But, right now, Rick has to take care of his family and his job."

"We understand," Wanda said gently. "We care about you, Rick, and we want what's best. Whatever path you take, we want you to know that healthy or unhealthy, you're our friend."

"Thanks," Rick said. He patted his belly fondly. "Then you'll understand why I have to be well before I can be a Wellness Wombat. I have to get out of the maze before I can guide others out of it, and that's going to take some time."

"But, if you repeat your unhealthy history you place a vote for medicine to repeat theirs."

"I know, Warren, I know. I appreciate the time you've taken to help me see how I got on this unhealthy path. I'm just not sure when I'll have time to take the first step to get off."

"While you're telling your friends about how you almost died in the medical maze, tell them about the alternative to that maze that we've shared with you," Ed suggested. "It may remind you to take some alternative steps yourself."

"Ed's right," Wanda said. "Your story may make others wary of being pulled into the same maze you narrowly escaped. They might even thank you, one day, for opening their eyes to alternatives, and for suggesting they learn to move their own magnets."

"I'll have to make some pretty big changes to move the people I know well enough to make them want to move their own magnets," Rick replied. "They'll have to see me much healthier before they question their ways and the maze those ways are leading them into."

"No one likes change, but change is what people are going to have to do," Warren said, sitting back up, "if they want to stay out of the medical maze. They must change the way they think about whose hands their health is in. They must embrace the Wellness Wombats and become educated about how to manage their own health and have fun doing it. They should look at how often the media is talking about the problems medicine is having and how much it costs to be sick today."

"And how much demand there is for alternative medicine," Doctor Ed added. "The people that medicine has been suppressing for so many years now want to suppress medicine. Now it is medicine's turn to be ridiculed, doubted, and questioned."

"You're right of course. The internet has made it possible for everyone to become better informed about how the medical maze works and better armed when they have to go in there." Warren looked at Rick again. "So your friends just might be better informed than you think. They might be frustrated, too, with how dependent they've been conditioned to become on medicine when they get sick."

"Help your friends," Ed pleaded, as he put his juice down. "Share The Five Ways to Stay out of the Maze card with them. Better yet, ask them to do what other concerned consumers do: protest Main Street's consuming ways by consuming less fast food."

"Yes," Warren said. "Help us flip that 'M' on Main Street to a 'W' for Wellness. Ooops. Sorry, Rick, I didn't explain this one to you did I? The 'M' stands for Main Street's fast food meat menus, an 'M' that we would all like to invert to a 'W' for Wellness based menus instead."

Rick grinned. "Like the menu here at Quackers, you mean?"

"You bet. Consumer eating habits are about as automated as the restaurants that grind out what those consumers eat,"

Warren protested. "That's why marketers call them consumers. If your friends quit eating in places that serve unhealthy foods, they will help themselves and their communities by flipping the Big M, archrival to the Big W, upside down. They'll help break the cycle that feeds you and your friends, just as though you were on a conveyor belt, right into the medical maze."

"They'll be Wellness Wombats without even realizing it," Wanda cheered enthusiastically, "boycotting not just one Burger Company, but all who in the name of serving billions do the nation's health a disservice."

"Boycotting Main Street isn't the goal," Warren quickly explained: "Getting people to respond to today's health trends and the wellness movement is."

"Don't look so worried, Rick," Ed said. "You can still eat out. You don't have to change that, just change the choices you make. Avoid artificial sweeteners, sodas, and processed foods. Ask about and demand healthier content. The health of the nation is at stake."

Rick shrugged. "You guys have big goals for a bunch of little ol' Wellness Wombats. I admire your vision: turning people's minds around about whose hands their health is in."

"It will happen, one Wellness Wombat at a time. We're optimistic. Wellness and environmental issues are penetrating every community these days," Warren said as he reached for his wallet. "Anyway, I believe that you were attracted to Quackers for a reason. And I hope that everything we've shared with you helps you get on the path to health that you are looking for."

Rick glanced at his watch. "I might surprise you one day. But, right now the best path I can get on is the path through the park. I need to digest what you've shared and I need to be on time for my appointment." He scooted his chair back as he got ready to leave. "I'm back to the medical maze, for what I hope will be the last cut."

"Last cut? What do you mean," Wanda asked, "not more surgery?"

"I'm afraid so," Rick said, despondently. "Despite all this talk about getting out of the maze, I have an appointment set for this afternoon in fact. I'm due at Hickory Clinic to discuss how another doctor is going to undo the blunder the last one made. They have to open me up and take the surgical sponge they left inside when they operated on me. It's not a good story. I didn't really even want to tell you about it."

"They left a sponge inside you?" Wanda gasped, incredulous.

"That's right. They said it happens all the time. Would you believe that?" Rick slid his credit card across the table.

Warren put his hand on top of Rick's. "Put it away. We're buying lunch today." Ed offered a supporting arm as Rick struggled to get up.

"Don't worry," Rick said as he slowly looked at his three friends. "I'm fine, tired, but fine. But I do have to go. Thank you for lunch. Oh, and thank you for helping me see who moved my magnet."

"Thank the Wellness Wombats," Warren said.

"They did make medicine's history interesting," Rick replied, as he shuffled his feet across the patio tile and stepped unsteadily past Doc's garden maze until its shadows completely consumed him.

Prognosis:

Three Years Later

RICK STEPPED CONFIDENTLY THROUGH THE ADJOINING DOOR between The Quackery Health Food Store and Quackers Juice Bar, a crumpled brown bag under his arm. "Good to see you, Doc," he said as he tucked his sunglasses into his golf shirt. "This place is packed."

Doc's hand shielded his eyes from the September sun reflecting off the surface of the bar. And he broke into a smile. "What can I say? Everyone's crackers for lunch at Quackers. It's like this every day now. Used to be I was hurting for business and the fast food joints had the crowds; now it's the other way around. Wellness menus rule Main Street." Doc reached over the bar and faked a punch toward Rick's absent belly. "And look at you. You're in great shape. About time!"

"Thanks. I got over my love affair with my car so I'm walking everywhere now. It's the trend these days, you know. I actually love the exercise. It keeps me and my back problem out of the medical maze."

"Was that you I saw in the park last week with your kids?"

"It sure was. We love this neighborhood. It's so full of other health-conscious people. I'm glad we moved here, but my wife, Rita Linn, is still adjusting though."

"Wives are always adjusting. So is America, to all these new health trends," Doc said over the sound of the blenders. "Can I get you something?"

"No thanks. I'll order at the table. I'm having lunch with the Wellness Wombats. We're celebrating. It's been three years since they challenged me to change my ways and get out of the maze. Well, I've changed and I'm here to tell them how I did it."

"Warren and Wanda are up in the balcony," Doc shouted over his shoulder, as he headed to the other side of the bar. "Good luck fighting your way through the crowd."

Rick walked past the mini-maze and wombat topiary dominating the now expanded, but still cozy, Juice Bar. He climbed the four steps to the mezzanine level. "Hi, guys," he said, setting his groceries down on the wooden floor.

Wanda leapt up with her slender arms stretched out for a hug. "Rick! You look great."

Warren shook Rick's hand vigorously. "Yes, look at you; quite a change from a daze in the maze to healthier ways and fresh off the golf course, too."

"Thanks guys, good to see you both again."

"So, how's your golf game these days?"

"Great, Warren, but my ball is too much like me, it follows an alternative path."

Wanda laughed. "We want to hear how you got on that path. We've not kept up with each other the way we should."

"We've all been busy," Rick replied. "And I've been busy adjusting to my new lifestyle. The cash settlement from the lawsuit that Rita Linn insisted I file against Hickory Clinic changed a lot of things. I've got a gym at home now and a personal trainer."

"Oh, yes. The settlement from the sponge they left in you three years ago," Warren said. "That whole ordeal must have been terrible."

"It sure was. So, what have you two been up to?" Rick asked.

"I'm still lobbying at The Capitol to protect people's rights to manage their own health," Warren responded. "The Charter Spa and Wellness Center has Wanda hopping so, to spend time together, we talk at schools, churches, longevity lodges, and the well-care centers that are popping up everywhere."

"We take the Wellness Wombats, of course," Wanda added, helping herself to some quack snacks from the tray on the table, "to remind people to spread the word about wellness and the fact that healthy habits can be fun, especially if they keep you out of the medical maze."

"So what have you got in the grocery bag?" Warren demanded, peering into the open topped sack. "I see organic wheat-free bread, organic Muesili, Medjool dates. You're shopping at The Quackery?"

"I buy organic for the kids and me now. We're determined to move our own magnets."

"And your wife, is she still skeptical?" Wanda asked sitting back down as Rick took the seat across from her.

"When I first started talking about Wellness Wombats three years ago she was. Now she eats organic with us sometimes and even sips on the vegetable juices we make. But she teases us about this holistic stuff. And we tease her back. We joke about her trips with her girlfriends to Main Street's all-you-can-eat buffet bars."

"She's still caught in the ways of the maze then?" Wanda said.

"She heads for the emergency room at the first sign of a sniffle or shake. And she'll take the antibiotics that her doctors prescribe before she'll try an alternative remedy."

Warren reached for his Krushed Kiwi Kahuna Juice. "She'll come around when she's ready. You can't make someone change against her will. Tell us about your daughter, Hillary, isn't it?"

"Yes," he said with a proud grin. "She's busy being a Wellness Wombat. It's because of her I'm here today."

"You said that when we spoke on the phone, but you never told me why," Wanda said.

"Because I spoke to Hillary before I spoke to Rita Linn when I left here three years ago. And Hillary told me the truth. She told me I'd gotten two warnings, one at Hickory Clinic, and the other at Quackers with you. She said that I had to act on both of them. She said I had to change."

"So you began to move your magnet?"

"It sounds cheesy but, yes, I took responsibility," Rick admitted. "Over time, I slowly learned how to exchange my unhealthy lifestyle for a healthier one."

"Nothing cheesy about it," Warren proclaimed. "You decided to scurry right out of the medical maze and get on the path we steered you toward. I'm impressed. You didn't hem and haw for long then? Or stay stuck in your skeptical ways after leaving here?"

"I sniffed around for alternatives to your alternatives at first, believe me," Rick admitted, "but saw none."

"So you had to take action?" Warren asked.

Rick's grin disappeared. "As much as my back hurt, I had to do something. I learned how to attract positive health habits and repel negative ones, if that's what you mean.

Change my old ways for new ones and wrestle with my conditioning, in the process."

"So you ran with my Wellness Wombat idea?"

"I did, and I ran for exercise, too. That's how I got in shape for golf and why I can sit in a chair without fidgeting from pain now. But it was the two stuffed magnet-clutching Wellness Wombats you sent me, a few months after our history of medicine chat, that got me and Hillary going. She took them to her friends at school and told them it was time they learned how to move their own magnets; time they practiced healthy ways to stay out of the maze or they'd end up in the hospital like her Dad."

"We wanted you to have some of the first ones Rick," Wanda said, full of energy. "Now, three years later and the Wellness Wombats are everywhere: on fridge magnets, bumper stickers, T-shirts, and in the children's books Warren keeps writing. Wellness Wombats are recognized, now, as a fun way to encourage children and their parents to practice positive health habits, eliminate negative ones, and stay out of the healthcare maze."

"Your Wellness Wombats were a quick hit when Hillary first took them to class three years ago. The kids were hearing it from their parents about the junk food they ate at school back then. Becoming a Wellness Wombat sounded like more fun than being labeled a health nut for eating your veggies and skipping the burgers and buns. After Hillary introduced them at school, it suddenly became cool to talk about eating right and being healthy. Cool to use healthy ways to stay out of the maze and get away from Main Street's ways. Cool to bring better food to school rather than eating what the cafeteria served, or what the vending machines stocked. Cool to be a Wellness Wombat.

"Hillary would wave your magnet-clutching wombats around whenever she shared the stories you told me about witches, woodcutters, gravediggers, and so on. The kids began to see how much medicine and the food and drug vending companies were influencing their health. A lot of them at Hillary's school caught on fast to the idea that they could influence their own health and the health of others instead, by choosing to become Wellness Wombats, moving their own magnets, and then sharing the benefits of those new practices with others."

Rick continued. "You didn't know how involved I was with my church, or with Boy Scouts, but when the parents of my church study class and my scout troop found out from their kids that Hillary was responsible for spreading the news about the Wellness Wombats and the move your own magnet idea, they begged to know more. The parents couldn't believe how much fun their kids were having learning about healthy ways out of the medical maze. The rest, as you know, is history. Your ideas about moving your magnet to stay out of the medical maze and using the Wellness Wombats to make the idea real came along at exactly the right time."

"I bet they were a welcome break from the stay off drugs talks kids were used to hearing," Warren said.

"They were," Rick said. "The magnet metaphor made sense to the kids. So did the idea of passing the message on. They snapped up the Wellness Wombats quicker than Doctor Ed could stitch a wound. Besides, it was a lot more fun for kids to listen to a couple of Wellness Wombats showing them how to stay out of the medical maze and away from Main Street's menus, than to listen to some adult lecture them."

"It's a lot easier to steer kids away from Main Street's 'M' for manufactured food chains, to the 'W' for whole food ones," Warren stressed, "when Wellness Wombats are asking them to bypass fast food now and avoid a bypass later."

Wanda agreed. "Parents are tired of seeing their children being consumed by the messages constantly being marketed to them, and by the maze of merchandise that fast food chains entice families into collecting with their meals. Wellness Wombats fill kids' minds with healthy ideas, so they'll stop filling their stomachs with unhealthy food. That's why the new "I like MOM" sticker is such a hit."

"It's a great acronym: I like Moving My Own Magnet," Rick said, grinning. "It helps kids recruit their moms into feeding them better so they won't get fed into the maze later."

"A maze that in spite of its claims about embracing alternative medicine, still discredits it," Wanda complained. "I don't think medicine is too excited about having Wellness Wombats take money out of its pockets by teaching people how to manage their own health. Medicine would rather see the wellness movement, and the Wellness Wombats that are accelerating it, repeat history by becoming history."

Warren turned on his deep stage voice to emphasize his point. "The Wellness Wombats have come a long way. And so have you, Rick Weaver. A long way from the guy I wanted to throttle when he first walked in to Quackers Juice Bar ridiculing everything about our alternative lifestyle."

"It seemed the natural thing to do then," Rick quipped.

"No, really; I'm impressed, not just with how much healthier you are, but with the impact you've had on your community," Warren said, resuming his natural voice. "You're right; we never knew how involved you were with kids. You've done more than just become a Wellness Wombat; you've done what the wombats at the Sydney rest stop did. They learned their lessons about the hazards of

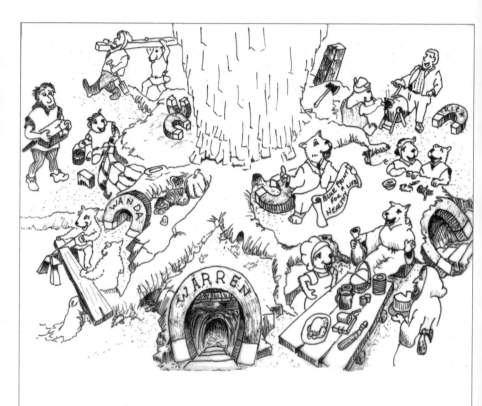

**Everybody helps his community
to weave a warren of wellness.**

manufactured food and led their warren, their community, down a healthier path."

"I think I've learned my lessons, too," Rick responded. "I didn't have time to get sick but I got sick anyway; from the fast food, fast acting medicine and fast answers I relied on to live my fast paced lifestyle. I was smart enough to slow down, but dumb enough to keep going, all the way to the hospital where I finally took the time to see how unhealthy the path I had taken was."

"Your story is as strong as any of the stories my Wellness Wombats told in the Ten Stages of medicine's history."

"It's a story that I weave into conversations with nearly everyone I meet these days: at home, at work, at church, at scouts, and even at baseball practice."

Warren raised his voice. "What did you say? Weaving? Wait. That's it! Rick Weaver the warren weaver. Every time you weave your story about your unhealthy journey into the maze and how we helped you out of it, you're helping to weave a warren of wellness into the community you share that story with."

"Rick Weaver the warren weaver?"

"Warren and Wanda Burrows talked to Rick Weaver about wellness. They inspired him to get well. He talked to people in his community about how good he felt and inspired others to get well, too. He became a Wellness Wombat but, more importantly, he became a warren weaver," Warren explained. "He wove warrens of wellness by inspiring others to pursue positive health habits; to walk the middle path to wellness and take care of themselves; not to depend on traditional or alternative medicine to do it for them."

"So a warren of wellness is where the people Wellness Wombats have influenced live, people eager to practice the ways that keep them out of the maze," Rick responded enthusiastically. "Warrens are everywhere then. In Atlanta, and all across the country."

Wanda looked perplexed. "So, a warren isn't just where wombats, or even rabbits, live?"

"No it's not," Warren chuckled. "A warren can be defined as a densely populated area: a place with a lot of winding streets, or hallways, a city, or even an apartment building. Atlanta is a warren, where carloads of unhealthy, overweight, overstressed, and over-medicated citizens weave their way through traffic listening to the news about our ongoing medical crisis. Rick is right. Atlanta, like every city, already has its warrens of wellness. Neighborhoods like ours have been warrens of wellness for years. Finally, more of them are sprouting up."

"I've been weaving warrens of wellness without knowing it then, haven't I? I live in one now." Rick nodded in approval. "I like it. The Wellness Wombats make the idea of an alternative lifestyle and sharing that lifestyle appealing, but your warren weaving idea invites people to do more. It invites them to contribute to the health of their community as well."

"Healthy citizens are the healthiest asset a country can have," Warren proclaimed.

"And your Wellness Wombats are bringing that movement to a boil, aren't they?"

"Yes," Warren said, "a boil that medicine keeps trying to lance."

"Wombats? Did I hear someone talking about wombats?"

"Ed!" Warren cried, looking up from his seat. "Sit down; we're ready to eat."

Rick reached out and shook Ed's hand. "Hello, Ed, it's great to see you."

Ed looked Rick up and down as he slid into the chair beside him. "You're looking well, my friend. And you've lost a notable amount of weight since I last saw you."

"I'll say. More than fifty pounds; and what have you been doing?"

"Recruiting doctors to come out of the medical maze, of course," Ed said. "Encouraging them to integrate alternative medicine and promote wellness instead of sickness. You'd be amazed how many are coming around. After reading the Wellness Wombats' rendition of their history they no longer feel compelled to protect it and are clamoring for a healthier medical model instead.

"I've been leveraging on the Wellness Wombats to help me flip Main Street's manufactured food menus to whole food menus, too, so that parents can choose restaurants that teach their kids good eating habits. I'm happy to say Hickory Clinic just canceled its contract with an onsite fast food company and brought in a whole foods chain instead, so that it can serve food that actually helps its patients to get well."

"Hillary's school kicked its vending machine company out and changed its school meals supplier," Rick said. "I think the skit the kids did for Wellness Week about wombats at a Sydney rest stop that got sick from eating the kind of food the school was feeding the kids may have had something to do with it."

Gaia appeared with her pad in her hand. "Hi there, Rick. Good to see you again. Are you folks ready to order yet?"

"Good to see you again, too, Gaia. Bring me a No GM juice, please and, in honor of our reunion, a Buffalo Burger and a Spinach Salad."

"That sounds good; I'll have the same," Warren said, "and another Kiwi Kahuna Juice."

"One more Green Piece Vicious Veggie, please," Wanda said, "with a Tofu and Turkey Sandwich."

Ed gave Gaia a warm smile. "A Chakra Corona Juice with a bowl of Pumpkin Soup."

"On its healthy way," Gaia said as she left.

So, how is that book of yours doing, Ed?" Rick asked. "What's it called, again?"

"It's called '*How Self-Care Contributes to our Nation's Healthcare.*' And thank you for asking. It's getting a lot of attention. But, that's not what we're here to celebrate, Rick. We all want to know why you're looking so good, and how you escaped the clutches of the medical maze by learning how to move your magnet. We could use your story in the ER Education Room, right Warren?"

"That's right, to arouse people to how their magnets are being moved and recruit more Wellness Wombats. Go ahead, Rick, tell us how you went from a daze in the maze to healthier days. We want to hear all about it."

"What were your first steps?" Wanda asked. "Did you use magnets, to stop your back from hurting?"

"I did and they helped. So did your Five Ways to Stay Out of the Maze checklist factors. I slept and exercised more, ate less, and reduced the amount of stress at work. I even told others about the middle path that you suggested: the 'Self-Care Is Better for You Than Healthcare,' one. I haven't been near the medical maze since they took that sponge out."

"That had to be a terrible experience. But this is exciting," Warren sympathized. "You've changed your mind, and your habits. Tell us more."

"I changed my mind because I realized it was time I returned it to its rightful owner and learned how to be my own guru. Not something society encourages, you know. I read health books, magazines, and Internet articles to learn more about my body. I paid attention to what my body was telling me. I stopped eating when my belly told me it was full. I quit working when I felt tired instead of pushing myself all the time and spent more time with my family." Rick started to grin. "I monitored my habits to see if they were negative or positive; if I was living like hell or living well."

"Acting less like the old sick Rick and more like a Wellness Wombat, you mean," Ed commented.

"We all stray from the path now and then," Wanda remarked. "The odd pizza now and then or party food we're sorry we fell for the morning after. But you stuck with it, Rick. You did what most people aren't willing to do. You invested in your own health."

"Don't make me out to be the hero," Rick answered. "I was stuck like a magnet to my unhealthy habits before you helped me pull away from them. It's because of you that I'm in the shape I'm in today. You showed me how much the medical maze influenced my thinking, and how duped I'd been. You forced me to ask questions about my health habits I'd been too busy or too lazy to entertain before. That's all."

"So our strategy worked; our Wellness Wombat stories got you to think."

"It wasn't easy, Warren, especially at work with my cable crews and office staff. It wasn't easy at home, either, with my wife and son calling Hillary and me health nuts and betting our new craze wouldn't last."

"Congratulations even more so on really sticking with it," Ed said wholeheartedly.

"It was easier with Hillary as my partner. We coached each other, so we could overcome our doubts about your Wellness Wombats and our fears about going alternative. Our friends and family ribbed us if we strayed off, or stayed on, the path. Our soda sipping, junk-food habits were not easy to break. The Five Ways checklist was a great guide, but it was Hillary's determination that got us through. She wanted other people to see what you two had shown me: how consumed we are by our unhealthy habits and the truth behind the medical maze that those habits feed us into."

"She's persistent. You both are," Wanda said. "So, did any of your family or friends come around?"

"They're beginning to," Rick replied. "My friends see me walking every day and they know that I spend more time with my kids. My family knows that what I'm doing now is healthier than anything I've ever tried before. And, more people want to know what I'm doing because I look so good well, healthy, I mean."

"We can see it in your face. You radiate health now," Wanda said with a happy smile. "Some of the people you know have come to my Spa and Wellness Center, and told me you sent them. I think they see that this wellness trend is here to stay."

"It's the way society is going," Rick replied. "Look at all the organic food chains, oxygen bars, nap centers, longevity lodges, and well-care centers on Main Street now. And how many offices and homes have air and water purifiers."

"People are nervous because the crutch they called health-care can't afford to provide the same services it used to," Warren warned. "Medicine expects them to take more responsibility for their health now."

"Employers do, too," Rick said firmly. "Most of them have cut back on health benefits and encourage their staff to focus on wellness instead. One of the posters at work sums up my boss's new philosophy. It says: 'The best health benefits you will receive are the ones you get from taking care of yourself.' Well, that's certainly something Hillary and I learned from you two. The first thing we did to take care of ourselves was to help each other get off Main Street. We both kept a personal checklist. Did we drive home to eat that day, or go through the drive-thru? Did I quit my donuts and coffee breakfast-in-the truck ritual and my drive-thru-between-meals habits? Did Hillary stop eating the junk Main Street fast food joints served when she hung out with her friends after school?"

"Did she?" Wanda asked.

"She did," Rick said proudly. "I quit eating at those places, too, as part of the last minute 'where shall we go eat lunch?' ritual at work. I ate the yeast free spelt bread sandwiches Hillary made for me instead. Eventually, we both got off Main Street's menus altogether and ate at home. We changed what we ate and how we ate. No more ordering pizza. No television during meals. No more answering our cell phones or hurrying away from the table with the last bites in our mouths. We actually talked to each other instead. Rita Linn liked that part best; in fact, we all did."

"Disciplines most people don't take time for today," Warren said, "especially the part about taking time to enjoy your meal and talk things over with friends and family."

"They'd gain time if they did. Lifetime, I mean. Those disciplines have given me a sense of well-being that I never had before. They helped me get my body to where it is today, so that I can walk back in here looking like this and show you guys I could do it. Besides, I'll have more choices later in life because of the changes I'm making now. Giving up soda for water, reducing my beer intake, and eliminating fast foods and sugar-filled desserts are small prices to pay for a longer life."

"Did Hillary break her snacking on junk food between meals habit?" Ed asked.

"She did. She bought dried fruit, organic trail mix, and other healthy stuff from The Quackery next door to snack on instead and kept it in her school bag." Rick gestured in the direction of Hickory Clinic. "We've both replaced our old ways with new ways, so we can stay out of the maze."

Rick looked at Warren for a moment. "You know, three years ago, I didn't even know I was caught up in the ways of that maze and the medical trap. Now I'm warning others about it, just like you warned me. It hasn't been easy to change my mind about who was responsible for my health. And, I can see why people let medicine, the food industry, and their jobs run their life. It is work getting out of the maze."

"Work that's paid off, though," Wanda said with a smirk on her face.

Rick patted his flat stomach. "Yeah, I know. I feel great. I would do it again if I had to. But I don't intend to, because I see a healthier future if I stay on this alternative path you all helped to put me on."

"A path that's more fun to walk when you've got the Wellness Wombats sharing the way," Ed said.

"If it hadn't been for Warren and Wanda, there wouldn't be any Wellness Wombats, my friend," Rick responded. "It's thanks to them that thousands of parents who wanted to live healthier lives and teach their kids to do the same have learned how to move their own magnets."

"And stay out of the maze other doctors call medicine," Ed added.

"I appreciate the credit that you're giving me, Rick," Warren said firmly. "But if Doc hadn't taught me what I know now when I walked into Quackers as one of his first customers twenty three years ago, we wouldn't even be talking about moving magnets or weaving warrens of wellness right now."

"I couldn't have opened my Spa without knowing what Doc taught me," Wanda added.

"I don't think this is about the difference Doc's made, Ed's made, you've made, or even that we've made, Rick," Warren said with a voice of authority. "It's about creating a healthier history for the next generation to hold on to and claim for their own instead of letting them repeat the unhealthy history of medicine's past. It's more about teaching people how to move their own magnets than it is about how medicine and the food and drug industry teach you to become a magnet attracted to the ways of the maze, the fast food trays and the medication haze."

"Then we have to depend on the power that the Wellness Wombats and their word of mouth strategy actually have to create warrens of wellness in every community and, in its wake, a healthier history of medicine," Rick said enthusiastically, "so that medicine's medical history will be something doctors can proudly share one day and not hide behind or mask over."

He suddenly looked over Warren's shoulder toward the front door and the others turned their heads, wondering what he was staring at so intently.

"Well I know who I'm going to help create a healthier history. See that overweight guy standing at the entrance? I've seen him before. I think he lives around here. But would you look at him now? He looks like he just got out of Hickory Clinic. In fact he still has his hospital tags on.

"That's a 'help me' look if ever I saw one," Rick said as he hurriedly jumped to his feet. "Stay put, guys; I'll be right back. And pull up another chair. Oh, and order another juice.

"I'm going to invite him to join us. Could be he wants to learn how to stay out of that medical maze and move his own magnet. And maybe even become a Wellness Wombat."

THE END

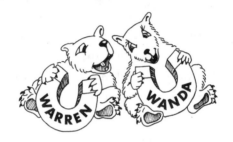

APPENDIX

Five Ways to Stay Out of the Maze and Move Your Own Magnet

Number one: Be conscious of what you are fed by the world, by food and drug companies, by medicine, and by media messiahs. Don't get drawn into their ways.

Number two: Respect your body and help it help itself by giving it the time and environment it needs every day to get regular exercise, proper nutrition, clean water, clean air, and sufficient sleep.

Number three: Go outside. Nurture your connection to nature. Listen to the rhythm and pulse of your body, and to your intuition. It will tell you what is good for you.

Number four: Address stress. Spend more time being still and less time being busy.

Number five: Walk the middle path to wellness; don't depend on alternative or traditional care. Self-care is better for you than the maze we call healthcare.

Four Questions to Ask if Your Doctor Invites You to Enter the Medical Maze

1) Am I attracted to or repelled by this aspect of healthcare?

2) Is it moving my magnet for me or is it helping me to move my own?

3) Does it support or repress my rights?

4) Does it help or hinder my ability to manage my own health?

Warren's Ten Stages Of Medicine's History In Which He Reveals The Ways Medicine Built Its Maze

1. **Gwen and Godfrey: The Witch and the Woodcutter:** How the power plays on which the foundations of the medical maze were built and how the hoax medicine played wrestled away the right people had to heal themselves.

2. **Mel and Matilda: The Guard at the Gate and the Cook Who Couldn't Wait:** How medicine minimized the validity of alternative natural medicine during its quest to secure trust, shake off its own quack label, and establish territory.

3. **Mort: Garlic for the Gravedigger:** How traditional medicine spawned Public Health Boards and medical schools to expand its influence, an important brick-laying phase in the construction of the maze.

4. **Heather and Horace: The Herb Lady's Potions and the Doctor's Lotions:** How the doctrine that medical schools taught and still pass down today was founded on how impressed medicine was by itself and its discoveries, and went like this: the human body is far too complex for people to heal; only medicine can manage the public's health now.

5. **Mason, Morgan, and Morris: The Bloodletter, the Body Snatcher and the Knife Grinder:** How the incision decision was made and surgery began.

6. **Florence: The Nurse at the Camp with a Swinging Lamp:** How medicine treated women and how one woman challenged its male dominated maze.

7. **Harvey: Red as Blood: White as Linen:** How medical men defended their position and the maze by building more walls in the form of Gentlemen's Clubs, Surgeons' Clubs, Guilds, and Medical Associations: all places where women were not admitted.

8. **Sherman: The Water Worker:** How public health lost control and medicine took control; and the people lost faith in the former and gained faith in the latter.

9. **Benjamin: The Doctor's Rush for a Healthy Constitution:** How the growth of medical colleges and schools was controlled and how the public became dependent upon medicine.

10. **Sheila: The Wide-Eyed Wombat:** How medicine consumed others with its quackery to draw them into its maze and cement itself in the minds of consumers.

REFERENCES AND SUGGESTED READING

Ausubel, K. *When Healing Becomes a Crime*. Rochester, VT: Healing Arts Press, 2000.

Bell, CM, Redelmeier, DA. *Mortality among Patients Admitted to Hospitals on Weekends as Compared with Weekdays*. N Engl J Med 345: 663-668.

Benyus, J. *Biomimicry: Innovation Inspired by Nature*. New York: Morrow, 1997.

Birla, GS, Hemlin, C. *Magnet Therapy. The Gentle and Effective Way to Balance Body Systems*. Rochester, VT: Healing Arts Press, 1999.

Bunch, B. *Handbook of Current Health & Medicine*. Pontiac: Gale Group, 1994.

Carlson, R. *The End of Medicine*. New York: John Wiley & Sons, 1975.

Carter, JP. *Racketeering in Medicine. The Suppression of Alternatives*. Norfolk: Hampton Roads, 1992.

Fraser, JA. *White-Collar Sweatshop*. New York: W.W. Norton, 2001.

Garrett, L. *Betrayal of Trust: The Collapse of Global Public Health*. New York: Hyperion, 2000.

Gladwell, M. *The Tipping Point. How Little Things Can Make a Big Difference*. Boston: Little, Brown, 2000.

Haley, D. *Politics in Healing*. Washington, DC: Potomac Valley Press, 2001.

Harris, M. *Cows, Pigs, Wars & Witches: The Riddles of Culture*. New York: Vintage Books, 1989.

Hayek, FA. *The Road to Serfdom*. Chicago: University of Chicago Press, 1944.

Johnson, P. *A History of the American People*. New York: Harper, 1997.

Johnson, P. *The Birth of the Modern: World Society, 1815-1830*. New York: Harper Collins, 1991.

Johnson, P. *Modern Times: The World from the Twenties to the Eighties*. New York: Harper Collins, 1983.

Johnson, S. *Who Moved my Cheese?* New York: G.P. Putnam's Sons, 1998.

Jacques Leslie, *Unsanitary Behavior.* Mother Jones, July/August 1997, p28.

Knowles, JH. *Doing Better and Feeling Worse: Health in the United States.* New York: Norton, 1977.

McDonough, W, Braungart, M. *The Next Industrial Revolution.* Atlantic Monthly, Oct 1998: 82-92.

Nash, RA. *Common Sense Medicine.* New York: iUniverse.com, 2000.

Payne, B. *The Body Magnetic.* Santa Cruz: Psychophysics, 1999.

Pilzer, PZ. *The Next Trillion.* Dallas: VideoPlus, 2001.

Porter, R. *The Greatest Benefit to Mankind: A Medical History of Humanity.* New York: W.W. Norton & Company, 1998.

Rock, A. *Is Your Hospital Gambling With Your Life?* Reader's Digest 2001.

Roizen, MF. *Real Age - Are You as Young as You Can Be?* New York: Harper Collins, 1999.

Toffler, A, Toffler, H. *Creating a New Civilization: The Politics of the Third Wave.* Atlanta: Turner Pub, 1995.

Whyte, D. *Crossing the Unknown Sea.* New York: Riverhead Books, 2001.

Williamson, M. *The Healing of America.* New York: Simon & Schuster, 1997.

Ordering Book Stacks and WELLNESS WOMBATS™
Spreading the word about wellness

Who Moved My Magnet? is $12.95 per copy
Add $5.50 shipping/handling for first two books
$3.00 each additional book (USA only)
(Currency exchange and additional postage fees will be applied to international orders)

Bulk order Discounts available when you buy stacks of books!
Go to www.whomovedmymagnet.com

Online orders: www.whomovedmymagnet.com

Postal orders: AMT ProduXions LLC
12460 Crabapple Road, Ste 202 # 377
Alpharetta, GA 30004

Phone orders: 1-888 WOMBAT1 (966 2281) Have your credit card ready.

Fax orders: 1-877 WOMBAT1 (966 2281) Fax in this completed form.

Name: _____

SHIPPING ADDRESS _____

City: _____ State: _____ Zip: _____

Email address: _____

Telephone: _____

Name: _____

BILLING ADDRESS (For credit card orders) _____

City: _____ State: _____ Zip: _____

Email address: _____

Telephone: _____

Qty. books _____ x $12.95 = _____ + S&H = _____ + tax 7% (GA) = _____
(Add S&H of $5.50 for first two books and $3.00 each additional book. USA only)

Payment: ❏ Check ❏ VISA ❏ MASTERCARD ❏ DISCOVER

Card number: _____

Name on card: _____ Exp. Date:_____/_____
For products shipped to Georgia ONLY please add 7% tax

Plush toy WELLNESS WOMBATS™ coming soon.

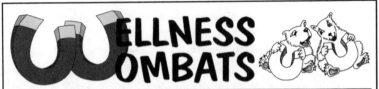

WELLNESS WOMBATS

Move their own magnets to stay out of the medical maze
www.whomovedmymagnet.com

Ordering Book Stacks and WELLNESS WOMBATS™
Spreading the word about wellness

Who Moved My Magnet? is $12.95 per copy
Add $5.50 shipping/handling for first two books
$3.00 each additional book (USA only)
(Currency exchange and additional postage fees will be applied to international orders)

Bulk order Discounts available when you buy stacks of books!
Go to www.whomovedmymagnet.com

Online orders: www.whomovedmymagnet.com

Postal orders: AMT ProduXions LLC
12460 Crabapple Road, Ste 202 # 377
Alpharetta, GA 30004

Phone orders: 1-888 WOMBAT1 (966 2281) Have your credit card ready.

Fax orders: 1-877 WOMBAT1 (966 2281) Fax in this completed form.

Name: _____

SHIPPING ADDRESS _____

City: _____ State: _____ Zip: _____

Email address: _____

Telephone: _____

Name: _____

BILLING ADDRESS (For credit card orders) _____

City: _____ State: _____ Zip: _____

Email address: _____

Telephone: _____

Qty. books _____ x $12.95 = _____ + S&H = _____ + tax 7% (GA) = _____
(Add S&H of $5.50 for first two books and $3.00 each additional book. USA only)

Payment: ❑ Check ❑ VISA ❑ MASTERCARD ❑ DISCOVER

Card number: _____

Name on card: _____ Exp. Date:_____/_____

For products shipped to Georgia ONLY please add 7% tax

Plush toy WELLNESS WOMBATS™ coming soon.

Find the WELLNESS WOMBATS™ Hidden in this puzzle.

```
R W H M O R E M B O L N U R S E M E

B A C D K O E X L E D M A S O N E N

N S Z A H C L H O R O D E N Q T C A

I T W N A A I Q T A N N W H R A A M

M A A N D N R R X A L Y A O Z F R R

A P R Y L I Y V W L E I M S M D O E

J H R D I N G O E Z K H E P E B H H

N O E S T E Q W N Y X D D H L Y A S

E A N R A F L O R E N C E L S O I T

B U G W M E Z A M O W N V G D R V G

R U V R I Y E R F D O G O E R P I L

D T W P O E N I C I D E M O S I C K

T E N G A M S W E L L T M B W E L L
```

WOMBAT	WELLNESS	WARREN	WANDA
RICK	ED	GWEN	GODFREY
MEL	MATILDA	MORT	MAGNET
MAZE	HEATHER	HORACE	MASON
MORRIS	FLORENCE	HARVEY	SHERMAN
DR. BENJAMIN	SHEILA	MOVED	MORGAN